BARBARA KRAUS
CALO... ...O
BRA... ...
AND BASIC FOODS

Contains hundreds of new entries including:

•

Little Caesar's, 7-Eleven, Pizza Hut
and Arthur Treacher's

•

Weight Watchers Ultimate 200 Meals

•

Dove Ice Cream bars

•

Budget Gourmet, Health Valley
and Ultra Slim Fast Foods

•

Chef America Lean Pockets

•

Alpine Lace Cheese

•

Famous Amos, Mother's and
Frookie Cookies and Crackers

•

Dunkin' Donuts

•

Simplesse Simple Pleasures Frozen Desserts

•

TCBY Yog-a-Bars

•

Selected Pathmark Regular and No Frills Foods

•

Pepperidge Farm Soups

BARBARA KRAUS CALORIE GUIDE TO BRAND NAMES AND BASIC FOODS

A SIGNET BOOK

For Bryan Allen Molina

SIGNET
Published by the Penguin Group
Penguin Books USA Inc., 375 Hudson Street,
New York, New York 10014, U.S.A.
Penguin Books Ltd, 27 Wrights Lane,
London W8 5TZ, England
Penguin Books Australia Ltd, Ringwood,
Victoria, Australia
Penguin Books Canada Ltd, 10 Alcorn Avenue,
Toronto, Ontario, Canada M4V 3B2
Penguin Books (N.Z.) Ltd, 182-190 Wairau Road,
Auckland 10, New Zealand

Penguin Books Ltd, Registered Offices:
Harmondsworth, Middlesex, England

First published by Signet, an imprint of Dutton Signet, a
division of Penguin Books USA Inc.

First Printing, January, 1994
10 9 8 7 6 5 4 3 2 1

 REGISTERED TRADEMARK–MARCA REGISTRADA

Printed in the United States of America

Foreword

The composition of the foods we eat is not static: it changes from time to time. In the case of *brand-name* products, manufacturers alter their recipes to reflect the availability of ingredients, advances in technology, or improvements in formulae. Each year new products appear on the market and some old ones are discontinued.

On the other hand, information on *basic foods* such as meats, vegetables, and fruits may also change as a result of the development of better analytical methods, different growing conditions, or new marketing practices. These changes, however, are usually relatively small as compared with those in manufactured products.

Some differences may be found between the values in this book and those appearing on the product labels. This is usually due to the fact that the Food and Drug Administration permits manufacturers to round the figures reported on labels. The data in this book are reported as calculated without rounding. If large differences between the two sets of values are noted, they may be due to changes in product formulae, and in those cases the label data should be used.

For all these reasons, a book of calorie or nutritive values of foods must be kept up to date by a periodic review and revision of the data presented.

Therefore, this handy calorie counter provides the most current and accurate estimates available. Generous use of this little book will help you and your family to select the right foods and the proper number of calories each member requires to gain, lose, or maintain healthy and attractive weight.

Why This Book?

Some of the data presented here can be found in more detail in my best-selling *Calories and Carbohydrates,* a dictionary of more than 8,000 brand names and basic foods. Complete as it is, it is meant to be used as a reference book at home or in the office.

Therefore, responding to the need for a portable calorie guide, and one which can reflect food changes often, I have written this smaller and handier version. The selection of material and the additional new entries provide readers with pertinent data on thousands of products that they would prepare at home to take to work, eat in a restaurant or luncheonette, nibble on from the coffee cart, take to the beach, buy in the candy store, et cetera.

For the sake of saving space and providing you with a greater selection of products, I had to make certain compromises: whereas in the giant book there are several physical descriptions of a product, here there is but one.

For Beginners Only

The language of dieting is no more difficult to learn than any other new subject; in many respects, it's much easier, particularly if you restrict your education to clearly defined goals.

For you who never before had the need or the interest in a lesson in weight control, I offer the following elementary introduction, applicable to any diet, self-initiated or suggested by your doctor, nutritionist, or dietician.

A Calorie

An analysis of foods in terms of calories is most often the chosen method to describe the relative energy yielded by foods.

A calorie is a shorthand way to summarize the units of energy contained in any foodstuff or alcoholic beverage, similar to the way a thermometer indicates heat. One pound of fat is equal to 3,500 calories. Add this number of calories to those you need to balance your energy requirements and you will gain one pound; subtract it and you will lose a pound.

Other Nutrients

Carbohydrates—which include sugars, starches, and acids—are only one of several chemical compounds in foods that yield calories. Proteins, found mainly in beef, poultry, and fish; fats, found in oils, butter, marbling of meat, and poultry skin; and alcohol, found in some beverages, also contribute calories. Except for alcohol, most foods contain at least some of these nutrients.

The amount of carbohydrates varies from zero in meats and a trace in alcohol to a heavy concentration in sugar, syrups, some fruits, grains, and root vegetables.

As of this date, the most respected nutritional researchers insist that a diet high in carbohydrates is necessary for maintaining good health. The amount to be included is an individual matter, and in any drastic effort to change your eating patterns, be sure to consult your doctor first.

Now, on how to use this new language.

To begin with, you use this book like a dictionary. If your plan is to cut down on calories, the easiest way to do so is to consult the portable calorie counter and keep an accurate count of your total intake of food and beverages for a period of seven days. If you have not gained or lost weight during that week, divide that number by seven and you'll have your maintenance diet expressed in calories. To lose weight, you must reduce your daily or weekly intake of calories below this maintenance level. (To gain, increase the intake.)

Keeping in mind that you want to stay healthy and eat well-balanced meals (which include the basic food groups—vegetables and fruits; whole grain or enriched breads, pastas, or cereal; fish, poultry, meat; milk or milk products; as well as some fats or oils), you then start to cut down on your portion in order to reduce your intake of calories. There are many imaginative ways to diet without total withdrawal from one's favorite foods.

Once you know and don't have to guess what calories are in your foods, you can relax and enjoy them. It could turn out that dieting isn't so bad after all.

ABBREVIATIONS AND SYMBOLS

*	= prepared as package directs[1]	oz.	= ounce
<	= less than	pkg.	= package
&	= and	pt.	= pint
"	= inch	qt.	= quart
canned	= bottles or jars as well as cans	T.	= tablespoon
dia.	= diameter	Tr.	= trace
fl.	= fluid	sq.	= square
liq.	= liquid	tsp.	= teaspoon
lb.	= pound	wt.	= weight
med.	= medium		

Italics or name in parentheses = registered trademark, ®. All data not identified by company or trademark are based on material obtained from the United States Departments of Agriculture or Health and Human Services (formerly Health, Education and Welfare)/Food and Agriculture Organization.

EQUIVALENTS

By Weight	By Volume
1 pound = 16 ounces	1 quart = 4 cups
1 ounce = 28.35 grams	1 cup = 8 fluid ounces
3.52 ounces = 100 grams	1 cup = ½ pint
	1 cup = 16 tablespoons
	2 tablespoons = 1 fluid ounce
	1 tablespoon = 3 teaspoons
	1 pound butter = 4 sticks or 2 cups

[1]If the package directions call for whole or skim milk, the data given here are for whole milk unless otherwise stated.

Food and Description	Measure or Quantity	Calories

A

ABALONE, canned	4 oz.	91
AC'CENT	¼ tsp.	3
AGNELOTTI, frozen (Buitoni):		
Cheese filled	2-oz. serving	196
Meat filled	2-oz. serving	206
ALBACORE, raw, meat only	4 oz.	201
ALLSPICE (French's)	1 tsp.	6
ALMOND:		
In shell	10 nuts	60
Shelled, raw, natural, with skins	1 oz.	170
Roasted, dry (Planters)	1 oz.	170
Roasted, honey (Eagle)	1 oz.	150
Roasted, oil (Tom's)	1 oz.	180
ALMOND BUTTER (Hain):		
Raw, natural	1 T.	95
Toasted, blanched	1 T.	105
ALMOND DELIGHT, cereal		
(Ralston Purina)	¾ cup (1 oz.)	110
ALMOND EXTRACT, pure		
(Durkee)	1 tsp.	13
ALPHA-BITS, cereal (Post)	1 cup (1 oz.)	110
AMARETTO DI SARONNO	1 fl. oz.	83
ANCHOVY, PICKLED, canned, flat or rolled, not heavily salted, drained		
(Granadaisa)	2-oz. can	80
ANISE EXTRACT, imitation		
(Durkee)	1 tsp.	16
ANISETTE:		
(DeKuyper)	1 fl. oz.	95
(Mr. Boston)	1 fl. oz.	88
APPLE:		
Fresh, with skin	2½" dia.	61
Fresh, without skin	2½" dia.	53
Canned:		
(Comstock):		
Rings, drained	1 ring	30
Sliced	⅙ of 21-oz. can	45

Food and Description	Measure or Quantity	Calories
(White House):		
Rings	1 ring	11
Sliced	½ cup (4 oz.)	54
Dried:		
(Sun-Maid/Sunsweet)	2-oz. serving	150
(Town House)	2-oz. serving	150
(Weight Watchers):		
Chips	¾-oz. pouch	70
Snack	.5-oz. pouch	50
Frozen, sweetened	1 cup	325
APPLE BROWN BETTY	1 cup	325
APPLE BUTTER:		
(Bama)	1 T.	36
(Empress)	1 T.	37
(Home Brands)	1 T.	52
(Smucker's)	1 T.	38
(White House)	1 T.	38
APPLE CHERRY BERRY DRINK,		
canned (Lincoln)	6 fl. oz.	90
APPLE CHERRY JUICE, canned		
(Red Cheek)	6 fl. oz.	113
APPLE CIDER:		
Canned:		
(Johanna Farms)	½ cup	56
(Musselman's) *Lucky Leaf*	6 fl. oz.	90
(Town House)	6 fl. oz.	90
(Tree Top)	6 fl. oz.	90
*Frozen (Tree Top)	6 fl. oz.	90
*Mix, *Country Time*	8 fl. oz.	98
APPLE CITRUS JUICE (Tree Top),		
canned or *frozen	6 fl. oz.	90
APPLE-CRANBERRY JUICE,		
canned (Lincoln)	6 fl. oz.	100
APPLE CRISP, frozen		
(Pepperidge Farm)	4¾ oz.	250
APPLE DRINK, canned:		
Capri Sun, natural	6¾ fl. oz.	90
Ssips (Johanna Farms)	8.45-fl.-oz. container	130
APPLE DUMPLINGS, frozen		
(Pepperidge Farm)	1 dumpling	260
APPLE, ESCALLOPED:		
Canned (White House)	½ cup (4.5 oz.)	163
Frozen (Stouffer's)	4 oz.	130
APPLE, GLAZED, frozen		
(Budget Gourmet) in raspberry		
sauce	5 oz.	110

Food and Description	Measure or Quantity	Calories
APPLE-GRAPE JUICE:		
Canned:		
(Mott's)	8.45-fl.-oz. container	128
(Red Cheek)	6 fl. oz.	109
(Tree Top)	6 fl. oz.	100
*Frozen (Tree Top)	6 fl. oz.	100
APPLE JACKS, cereal (Kellogg's)	1 cup (1 oz.)	110
APPLE JAM (Smucker's)	1 T.	53
APPLE JELLY:		
Sweetened:		
(Bama)	1 T.	45
(Empress)	1 T.	52
(Home Brands)	1 T.	52
(Smucker's)	1 T.	54
Dietetic:		
(Estee; Featherweight; Louis Sherry)	1 T.	6
(Diet Delight)	1 T.	12
(Pritikin)	1 T.	42
APPLE JUICE:		
Canned:		
(Borden) *Sippin' Pak*	8.45-fl.-oz. container	110
(Johanna Farms) *Tree Ripe*	8.45-fl.-oz. container	121
(Land O'Lakes)	6 fl. oz.	90
(Minute Maid)	6 fl. oz.	100
(Mott's)	6 fl. oz.	88
(Ocean Spray)	6 fl. oz.	90
(Red Cheek)	6 fl. oz.	85
(Town House)	6 fl. oz.	90
(Tree Top) regular	6 fl. oz.	90
(White House)	6 fl. oz.	87
Chilled (Minute Maid)	6 fl. oz.	91
*Frozen:		
(Minute Maid)	6 fl. oz.	91
(Sunkist)	6 fl. oz.	59
(Tree Top)	6 fl. oz.	90
APPLE JUICE DRINK, canned:		
Squeezit (General Mills)	6¾-oz. bottle	110
(Sunkist)	8.5 fl. oz.	140
APPLE NECTAR, canned (Libby's)	6 fl. oz.	100
APPLE PEAR JUICE, canned or *frozen (Tree Top)	6 fl. oz.	90

Food and Description	Measure or Quantity	Calories
APPLE PIE (See PIE, Apple)		
APPLE RAISIN CRISP, cereal (Kellogg's)	⅔ cup	130
APPLE RASPBERRY DRINK, canned (Mott's)	10-fl.-oz. container	158
APPLE RASPBERRY JUICE:		
Canned, regular pack:		
(Mott's)	8.45-fl.-oz. container	124
(Red Cheek)	6 fl. oz.	113
(Tree Top)	6 fl. oz.	80
*Frozen (Tree Top)	6 fl. oz.	80
APPLE-RASPBERRY JUICE COCKTAIL (Veryfine)	8 fl.oz.	110
APPLE SAUCE:		
Regular:		
(Hunt's) *Snack Pak:*		
Regular	4¼ oz.	50
Raspberry	4¼ oz.	80
(Mott's):		
Regular, jarred:		
Regular	6 oz.	150
Cinnamon	6 oz.	152
Single-serve cups:		
Regular	4 oz.	100
Cherry	3¾ oz.	72
Peach	3¾ oz.	75
Strawberry	3¾ oz.	76
(Town House)	½ cup	85
(Tree Top) original	½ cup	80
(White House) regular or chunky	½ cup	80
Dietetic:		
(Country Pure)	4 oz.	50
(Mott's) single-serve cups	4 oz.	53
(S&W) *Nutradiet,* white or blue label	½ cup	55
(Thank You Brand)	½ cup	54
(White House)	½ cup	50
APPLE STRUDEL, frozen (Pepperidge Farm)	3 oz.	240
APRICOT:		
Fresh, whole	1 apricot	18
Canned, regular pack:		
(Del Monte) whole, or halves, peeled	½ cup	100
(Stokely-Van Camp)	1 cup	220
(Town House) unpeeled, halves	½ cup	110

Food and Description	Measure or Quantity	Calories
Canned, dietetic, solids & liq.:		
(Country Pure) halves	½ cup	60
(Diet Delight):		
Juice pack	½ cup	60
Water pack	½ cup	35
(Featherweight):		
Juice pack	½ cup	50
Water pack	½ cup	35
(Libby's) Lite	½ cup	60
(S&W) *Nutradiet:*		
Halves, white or blue label	½ cup	50
Whole, juice	½ cup	40
Dried (Town House)	2 oz.	140
APRICOT LIQUEUR (DeKuyper)	1 fl. oz.	82
APRICOT NECTAR:		
(Ardmore Farms)	6 oz.	94
(Libby's)	6 fl. oz.	110
(Town House)	6 fl. oz.	100
APRICOT PRESERVE:		
Sweetened (Home Brands)	1 T.	51
Dietetic (Estee)	1 T.	6
APRICOT-PINEAPPLE NECTAR, canned, dietetic (S&W) *Nutradiet,* blue label	6 oz.	35
APRICOT & PINEAPPLE PRESERVE OR JAM:		
Sweetened:		
(Empress)	1 T.	52
(Home Brands)	1 T.	52
(Smucker's)	1 T.	53
Dietetic:		
(Diet Delight; Louis Sherry)	1 T.	6
(S&W) *Nutradiet*	1 T.	12
ARBY'S RESTAURANT:		
Bac'n Cheddar Deluxe	1 sandwich	510
Beef & Cheddar Sandwich	1 sandwich	500
Cake, cheese	3-oz. piece	305
Chicken breast sandwich	7¼-oz. sandwich	592
Croissant:		
Bacon & egg	1 croissant	430
Butter	1 croissant	260
Ham & swiss	1 croissant	340
Mushroom & swiss	1 croissant	340
Sausage & egg	1 croissant	520
French fries	2-oz. serving	245
Ham 'N Cheese	1 sandwich	330

Food and Description	Measure or Quantity	Calories
Potato cakes	2 pieces	201
Potato, stuffed:		
Broccoli & cheddar	1 potato	417
Deluxe	1 potato	620
Mushroom & cheese	1 potato	515
Roast beef:		
Regular	5 oz.	353
Junior	3 oz.	218
Super	9¼ oz.	530
Crackers	1 packet	25
Croutons	1 packet	70
Salads:		
Chef's (no dressing)	1 serving	235
Cashew chicken (contains dressing)	1 serving	590
Garden (no dressing)	1 serving	165
Salad dressings:		
Blue cheese	1 packet	295
Buttermilk	1 packet	350
Honey French	1 packet	320
Light Italian	1 packet	25
Soup:		
Cheese, Wisconsin	8 oz.	285
Chowder		
Clam, Boston	8 oz.	205
Corn, Pilgrim's	8 oz.	190
Tomato Florentine	8 oz.	85
ARTHUR TREACHER'S RESTAURANT:		
Chicken		
Patty	1 piece	184
Sandwich	5½ oz.	413
Chips	1 serv.	276
Cod Tail Shape	5 oz.	245
Coleslaw	3 oz.	123
Fish	1 piece	177
Fish sandwich	1 sandwich	440
Krunch Pup	2-oz. piece	203
Lemon Luv	3-oz. piece	276
Shrimp	7 pieces	381
ARTICHOKE:		
Boiled	15-oz. artichoke	187
Canned (Cara Mia) marinated, drained	6-oz. jar	175
Frozen (Birds Eye) deluxe	3 oz.	33

Food and Description	Measure or Quantity	Calories
ASPARAGUS:		
Boiled	1 spear (½" dia. at base)	3
Canned, regular pack, solid & liq.:		
(Del Monte) spears, green or white	½ cup	20
(Green Giant)	½ cup	20
(Town House) cut or whole	½ cup	20
Canned, dietetic, solids & liq.:		
(Diet Delight)	½ cup	16
(Featherweight) cut spears	1 cup	40
(S&W) *Nutradiet*	1 cup	40
Frozen:		
(Birds Eye):		
Cuts	⅓ pkg.	22
Spears	⅓ pkg.	23
(Frosty Acres)	3.3 oz.	25
(McKenzie)	⅓ pkg.	25
(Stouffer's) souffle	⅓ pkg.	115
ASPARAGUS PILAF, frozen (Green Giant) microwave *Garden Gourmet*	9½-oz. pkg.	190
ASPARAGUS PUREE, canned (Larsen)	½ cup	22
AUNT JEMIMA SYRUP (See SYRUP)		
AVOCADO (Calavo)	½ fruit, edible portion (3.05 oz.)	155
AVOCADO PUREE (Calavo)	½ cup (8.1 oz.)	411
***AWAKE* (Birds Eye)	6 fl. oz.	84

Food and Description	Measure or Quantity	Calories

B

BACON, broiled:
(Hormel) *Black Label*	1 slice	30
(Oscar Mayer):		
Regular slice	6-gram slice	35
Center cut	1 slice	25
Thick slice	1 slice	64

BACON, CANADIAN, unheated:
(Eckrich)	1 oz.	35
(Hormel):		
Regular	1 slice	45
Light & Lean ·	1 slice	17
(Oscar Mayer) 93% fat free:		
Thin	.7-oz. slice	30
Thick	1-oz. slice	35

BACON, SIMULATED, cooked:
(Oscar Mayer) *Lean'N Tasty*:		
Beef	1 strip	48
Pork	1 strip	54
(Swift's) *Sizzlean*:		
Beef	1 strip	35
Pork	1 strip	45

BACON BITS:
Bac*Os (Betty Crocker)	1 tsp.	12
(French's) imitation	1 tsp.	6
(Hormel)	1 tsp.	10
(Libby's) crumbles	1 tsp.	8
(Oscar Mayer) real	1 tsp.	6

BACON, TURKEY, cooked (Louis
Rich)	1 strip	32

BAGEL (Lender's):
Plain:		
Regular	1 bagel	150
Bagelette	1 bagel	70
Egg	1 bagel	150
Onion	1 bagel	160
Poppy seed	1 bagel	160
Raisin & honey	1 bagel	200

BAKING POWDER:
(Calumet)	1 tsp.	2

Food and Description	Measure or Quantity	Calories
(Davis)	1 tsp.	7
(Featherweight) low sodium, cereal free	1 tsp.	8
BAMBOO SHOOTS:		
Raw, trimmed	4 oz.	31
Canned, drained (Chun King)	½ cup	32
BANANA, raw (Dole)	6.3-oz. banana (weighed unpeeled)	101
BANANA EXTRACT, imitation (Durkee)	1 tsp.	15
BANANA NECTAR (Libby's)	6 fl. oz.	110
BANANA PIE (See PIE, Banana)		
BARBECUE SEASONING (French's)	1 tsp.	6
BARBERA WINE (Louis M. Martini) 12½% alcohol	3 fl. oz.	60
BARLEY, pearled (Quaker Scotch)	¼ cup	172
BASIL (French's)	1 tsp.	3
BASS:		
Baked, stuffed	3½" 4½" 1½"	531
Oven-fried	8¾" 4½" ⅝"	392
BATMAN, cereal (Ralston Purina)	1 cup	110
BAY LEAF (French's)	1 tsp.	5
B & B **LIQUEUR**	1 fl. oz.	94
B.B.Q. SAUCE & BEEF, frozen (Banquet) *Cookin' Bag,* sliced	4-oz. serving	100
BEAN, BAKED:		
(USDA):		
With pork & molasses sauce	1 cup	382
With pork & tomato sauce	1 cup	311
Canned:		
(Allen's) *Wagon Master*	1 cup	260
(B&M) *Brick Oven:*		
Pea bean with pork in brown sugar sauce	8 oz.	300
Red kidney bean in brown sugar sauce	8 oz.	290
Vegetarian	8 oz.	250
(Campbell's):		
Barbecue	7⅞-oz. can	210
Home style	8-oz. can	220
With pork & tomato sauce	8-oz. can	200
(Friend's):		
Pea	9-oz. serving	360
Yellow eye	9-oz. serving	360

Food and Description	Measure or Quantity	Calories
(Furman's) & pork, in tomato sauce	8 oz.	245
(Grandma Brown's)	8 oz.	289
(Health Valley):		
Boston, no salt added	½ cup	213
Vegetarian, with miso	½ cup	90
(Hormel) *Short Orders,* with bacon	7½-oz. can	330
(Hunt's) & pork	8 oz.	280
(Pathmark) in tomato sauce:		
Regular	½ cup	150
No Frills	½ cup	160
(Town House) & pork	1 cup	260
BEAN, BLACK OR BROWN:		
Dry	1 cup	678
Canned:		
(Goya)	½ cup	125
(Progresso)	½ cup	90
BEAN, CHILI, canned (Hunt's)	½ cup	90
BEAN, FAVA, canned (Progresso)	4 oz.	90
BEAN, GARBANZO, canned:		
Regular (Old El Paso)	½ cup	190
Dietetic (S&W) *Nutradiet,* low sodium, green label	½ cup	100
BEAN, GREEN:		
Boiled, 1½" to 2" pieces, drained	½ cup	17
Canned, regular pack, solids & liq.:		
(Allen's):		
Whole	½ cup	21
With dry shelled beans	½ cup	40
(A&P) cut	½ cup	20
(Green Giant) french or whole	½ cup	20
(Larsen) *Freshlike*	½ cup	20
(Pathmark):		
Regular, Blue Lake	½ cup	20
No Frills, cut	½ cup	18
(Town House) cut or french style	½ cup	20
Canned, dietetic, solids & liq.:		
(Del Monte) No Salt Added	4 oz.	19
(Diet Delight; S&W, *Nutradiet*)	½ cup	20
(Larsen) *Fresh-Lite*	½ cup	20
(Pathmark) no salt added	½ cup	20
Frozen:		
(A&P) cut or French style	3 oz.	25
(Bel-Air):		

Food and Description	Measure or Quantity	Calories
Cut or whole	3 oz.	25
With toasted almonds	3 oz.	45
(Birds Eye):		
Cut or french	⅓ pkg.	25
French, with almonds	3 oz.	52
Whole, deluxe	3 oz.	23
(Frosty Acres)	3 oz.	30
(Green Giant):		
Cut or french, with butter sauce, regular	3 oz.	30
Cut, *Harvest Fresh*	⅓ of 8-oz. pkg.	16
(Larsen)	3 oz.	25
(Seabrook Farms)	⅓ of 9-oz. pkg.	25
BEAN, GREEN & MUSHROOM CASSEROLE (Stouffer's)	½ of 9½-oz. pkg.	160
BEAN, GREEN, WITH POTATOES, canned (Sunshine) solids & liq.	½ cup	34
BEAN, ITALIAN:		
Canned (Del Monte) solids & liq.	4 oz.	25
Frozen:		
(Birds Eye)	3 oz.	31
(Frosty Acres; Larsen)	3 oz.	30
BEAN, KIDNEY:		
Canned, regular pack, solids & liq.:		
(Allen's) red	½ cup	110
(Furman) red, fancy, light	½ cup	121
(Goya):		
Red	½ cup	115
White	½ cup	100
(Hunt's):		
Regular	4 oz.	100
Small, red	½ cup (3.5 oz.)	90
(Progresso)	½ cup	100
(Town House) red	½ cup	110
Canned, dietetic (S&W) *Nutradiet,* low sodium	½ cup	90
BEAN, LIMA:		
Boiled, drained	½ cup	94
Canned, regular pack, solids & liq.:		
(Allen's):		
Regular	½ cup	60
Baby butter	½ cup	55
(Furman's)	½ cup	92
(Larsen) *Freshlike*	½ cup	80
(Sultana) butter bean	¼ of 15-oz. can	82

Food and Description	Measure or Quantity	Calories
(Town House) butter	½ cup	100
Canned, dietetic (Featherweight)	½ cup	80
Frozen:		
(Bel-Air) baby	3.3 oz.	130
(Birds Eye) baby	⅓ pkg.	126
(Frosty Acres):		
Baby	3.3 oz.	130
Butter	3.2 oz.	140
Fordhook	3.3 oz.	100
(Green Giant):		
In butter sauce	3.3 oz	83
Harvest Fresh	3 oz.	60
(Larsen) baby	3.3 oz.	130
(Seabrook Farms):		
Baby lima	⅓ of 10-oz. pkg.	126
Baby butter bean	⅓ of 10-oz. pkg.	139
Fordhook	⅓ of 10-oz. pkg.	98
BEAN, MEXICAN, canned		
(Old El Paso)	½ cup	163
BEAN, PINK, canned		
(Goya)	½ cup	115
BEAN, PINTO:		
Canned, regular pack, solids & liq.:		
(Gebhardt)	⅓ of 15-oz. can	245
(Goya) regular	½ cup (4 oz.)	100
(Green Giant)	½ cup	100
(Old El Paso)	½ cup	100
(Progresso)	½ cup	110
Frozen (McKenzie)	3.2-oz. serving	160
BEAN, RED, canned		
(Goya) small	½ cup	78
BEAN, REFRIED, canned:		
(Gebhardt) regular	4 oz.	130
Little Pancho, & green chili	½ cup	80
(Old El Paso):		
Plain	½ cup	110
With bacon	½ cup	208
With green chilis	½ cup	98
With sausage	½ cup	360
Vegetarian	½ cup	140
(Rosarita):		
Regular	4 oz.	130
With green chilis	4 oz.	116
Spicy	½ cup	120
Vegetarian	½ cup	120
BEAN, ROMAN, canned:		
(Goya)	½ cup	81

Food and Description	Measure or Quantity	Calories
(Progresso)	½ cup	110
BEAN, WHITE, canned		
(Goya) solids & liq.	½ cup	105
BEAN, YELLOW OR WAX:		
Boiled, 1" pieces, drained	½ cup	18
Canned, regular pack, solids & liq.:		
(Del Monte) cut or french	½ cup	18
(Larsen) *Freshlike*	½ cup	25
(Libby's) cut	4 oz.	23
(Stokely-Van Camp)	½ cup	23
Canned, dietetic (Featherweight)		
cut, solids & liq.	½ cup	25
Frozen (Frosty Acres)	3 oz.	25
BEAN & BEEF BURRITO		
DINNER, frozen (Swanson)	15¼-oz. dinner	720
BEAN & FRANKFURTER, canned:		
(Campbell's) in tomato and		
molasses sauce	7⅞-oz. can	360
(Hormel) *Short Orders,* 'n wieners	7½-oz. can	280
BEAN & FRANKFURTER		
DINNER, frozen:		
(Banquet)	10-oz. dinner	520
(Morton)	10-oz. dinner	350
(Swanson)	10½-oz. dinner	440
BEAN SALAD, canned		
(Green Giant)	½ cup	70
BEANS 'N FIXIN'S, canned (Hunt's)		
Big John's:		
Beans	3 oz.	100
Fixin's	1 oz.	50
BEAN SOUP (See SOUP, Bean)		
BEAN SPROUT:		
Mung, raw	½ lb.	80
Mung, boiled, drained	¼ lb.	32
Soy, raw	½ lb.	104
Soy, boiled, drained	¼ lb.	43
Canned (drained)	⅔ cup	6
BEAR CLAWS (Dolly Madison)		
cherry	2¾-oz. piece	270
BEEF, choice grade, medium done:		
Brisket, braised:		
Lean & fat	3 oz.	350
Lean only	3 oz.	189
Chuck, pot roast:		
Lean & fat	3 oz.	278
Lean only	3 oz.	182
Fat, separated, cooked	1 oz.	207

Food and Description	Measure or Quantity	Calories
Filet mignon (See Steak, sirloin, lean)		
Flank, braised, 100% lean	3 oz.	167
Ground:		
Regular, raw	½ cup	303
Regular, broiled	3 oz.	243
Lean, broiled	3 oz.	186
Rib:		
Roasted, lean & fat	3 oz.	374
Lean only	3 oz.	205
Round:		
Broiled, lean & fat	3 oz.	222
Lean only	3 oz.	161
Rump:		
Broiled, lean & fat	3 oz.	295
Lean only	3 oz.	177
Steak, club, broiled:		
One 8-oz. steak (weighed without bone before cooking) will give you:		
Lean & fat	5.9 oz.	754
Lean only	3.4 oz.	234
Steak, porterhouse, broiled:		
One 16-oz. steak (weighed with bone before cooking) will give you:		
Lean & fat	10.2 oz.	1339
Lean only	5.9 oz.	372
Steak, ribeye, broiled:		
One 10-oz. steak (weighed without bone before cooking) will give you		
Lean & fat	7.3 oz.	911
Lean only	3.8 oz.	258
Steak, sirloin, double-bone, broiled:		
One 12-oz. steak (weighed with bone before cooking) will give you:		
Lean & fat	6.6 oz.	767
Lean only	4.4 oz.	268
One 16-oz. steak (weighed with bone before cooking) will give you:		
Lean & fat	8.9 oz.	1028
Lean only	5.9 oz.	359

Food and Description	Measure or Quantity	Calories
Steak, T-bone, broiled:		
One 16-oz. steak (weighed with bone before cooking) will give you:		
Lean & fat	9.8 oz.	1315
Lean only	5.5 oz.	348
BEEF BOUILLON:		
Regular:		
(Herb-Ox):		
Cube	1 cube	6
Packet	1 packet	8
(Knorr)	1 cube	15
(Wyler's)	1 cube	6
Low sodium:		
(Borden) *Lite-Line*, instant	1 tsp.	12
(Featherweight)	1 tsp.	18
BEEF, CHIPPED:		
Cooked, home recipe	½ cup	188
Frozen, creamed:		
(Banquet)	4-oz. pkg.	100
(Stouffer's)	5½-oz. serving	230
BEEF DINNER OR ENTREE:		
*Canned:		
(Hormel) *Top Shelf*, roast, tender	1 serving	240
(Hunt's) *Entree Maker*, oriental	7.6 oz.	271
Frozen:		
(Armour):		
Classics Lite, Steak Diane	10-oz. meal	290
Dinner Classics, sirloin tips	10¼-oz. dinner	230
(Banquet):		
Dinner chopped	11-oz. dinner	420
Extra Helping	16-oz. dinner	870
Platter	10-oz. meal	460
Budget Gourmet, sirloin:		
Regular:		
Dinner, Three Dish, tips in burgundy sauce	11-oz. meal	310
Entree, tips, with country style vegetables	10-oz. meal	310
Light Entrees, in herb sauce	9½-oz. meal	270
Light & Healthy:		
Sliced in wine	11-oz. meal	270
Special recipe	11-oz. meal	250
Slim Selects, in herb sauce	9½-oz. meal	270
(Healthy Choice) sirloin tips	11⅜-oz. meal	290

Food and Description	Measure or Quantity	Calories
(La Choy) *Fresh & Lite*, & broccoli with rice	11-oz. meal	260
(Le Menu):		
Chopped sirloin	12¼-oz. dinner	430
Sirloin tips	11½-oz. dinner	400
Yankee pot roast	11-oz. dinner	360
(Morton) sliced	10-oz. dinner	220
(Stouffer's):		
Lean Cuisine, oriental with vegetables & rice	8⅝-oz. meal	250
Right Course:		
Dijon	9½-oz. meal	290
Fiesta	8⅞-oz. meal	270
(Swanson):		
Regular, 4-compartment, chopped sirloin	10¾-oz. dinner	340
Hungry Man:		
Chopped	16¾-oz. dinner	640
Sliced	15¼-oz. dinner	450
(Tyson) beef champignon	10½-oz. meal	370
(Weight Watchers):		
Stir fry:		
Cantonese	9-oz. meal	200
Jade Garden	9-oz. meal	150
Ultimate 200:		
London broil	7½-oz. meal	110
Sirloin tips	7½-oz. meal	200
BEEF, DRIED, canned:		
(Hormel)	1 oz.	45
(Swift)	1 oz.	47
BEEF GOULASH (Hormel)		
Short Orders	7½-oz. can	230
BEEF, GROUND, SEASONING MIX:		
*(Durkee):		
Regular	1 cup	653
With onion	1 cup	659
(French's) with onion	1⅛-oz. pkg.	100
BEEF HASH, ROAST:		
Canned, *Mary Kitchen* (Hormel):		
Regular	7½-oz. serving	350
Short Orders	7½-oz. can	360
Frozen (Stouffer's)	10-oz. meal	380
BEEF, PACKAGED		
(Carl Buddig)	1 oz.	40

Food and Description	Measure or Quantity	Calories
BEEF, PEPPER ORIENTAL,		
frozen:		
(Chun King)	13-oz. meal	310
(La Choy) dinner	12-oz. dinner	250
BEEF PIE, frozen:		
(Banquet)	7-oz. pie	510
(Empire Kosher)	8-oz. pie	540
(Morton)	7-oz. pie	430
(Swanson):		
Regular	7-oz. pie	370
Hungry Man	16-oz. pie	610
BEEF PUFFS, frozen (Durkee)	1 piece	47
BEEF ROLL (Hormel) Lumberjack	1 oz.	101
BEEF, SHORT RIBS, frozen:		
(Armour) *Dinner Classics,*		
boneless	9¾-oz. dinner	380
(Stouffer's) boneless, with gravy	9-oz. pkg.	350
BEEF SOUP (See SOUP, Beef)		
BEEF SPREAD, ROAST, canned		
(Underwood)	½ of 4¾-oz. can	140
BEEF STEAK, BREADED		
(Hormel) frozen	4-oz. serving	370
BEEF STEW:		
Home recipe, made with lean beef		
chuck	1 cup	218
Canned, regular pack:		
Dinty Moore (Hormel):		
Regular	8-oz. serving	210
Short Orders	7½-oz. can	150
(Libby's)	7½-oz. serving	170
(Nalley's) homestyle	8-oz. serving	180
(Pathmark) No Frills	8-oz. serving	190
Canned, dietetic:		
(Estee)	7½ oz.	210
(Healthy Choice)	7½ oz.	140
Frozen:		
(Banquet)	¼ of 28-oz. pkg.	140
(Freezer Queen) Family Supper	7 oz.	150
(Stouffer's)	10-oz. serving	305
Mix (Lipton)		
Microeasy, hearty	¼ pkg.	70
BEEF STEW SEASONING MIX:		
*(Durkee)	1 cup	379
(French's)	1 pkg.	150
BEEF STOCK BASE (French's)	1 tsp.	8
BEEF STROGANOFF, frozen:		
(Budget Gourmet) *Slim Selects*	8¾ oz. meal	280

Food and Description	Measure or Quantity	Calories
(Le Menu)	10-oz. dinner	430
(Stouffer's) with parsley noodles	9¾ oz.	390
(Weight Watchers)	9-oz. meal	320
*BEEF STROGANOFF SEASONING MIX (Durkee)	1 cup	820
BEEFAMATO COCKTAIL, canned		
(Mott's)	6 fl. oz.	80
BEER & ALE:		
Regular:		
Anheuser	8 fl. oz.	139
Black Horse Ale	8 fl. oz.	108
Black Label (Heilemann)	8 fl. oz.	68
Blatz (Heilemann)	8 fl. oz.	93
Budweiser	8 fl. oz.	118
Carlsberg	8 fl. oz.	100
Michelob, regular	8 fl. oz.	113
Old Milwaukee	8 fl. oz.	95
Pearl Premium	8 fl. oz.	99
Schlitz	8 fl. oz.	100
Stroh Bohemian	8 fl. oz.	84
Light or low carbohydrate:		
Bud Dry	8 fl. oz.	87
Budweiser, light	8 fl. oz.	73
Busch, light	8 fl. oz.	73
Carlsberg, light	8 fl. oz.	73
C. Schmidt's, light	8 fl. oz.	64
LA	8 fl. oz.	75
Michelob, dry	8 fl. oz.	88
Natural Light	8 fl. oz.	73
Special Export Light	8 fl. oz.	76
BEER BATTER MIX (Golden Dipt)	1 oz.	100
BEER, NEAR:		
Goetz Pale	8 fl. oz.	53
(Metbrew)	8 fl. oz.	49
BEET:		
Boiled, whole	2"-dia. beet	16
Boiled, sliced	½ cup	33
Canned, regular pack, solids & liq.:		
(Blue Boy) Harvard	½ cup	100
(Greenwood):		
Harvard	½ cup	70
Pickled	½ cup	110
(Larsen) *Freshlike:*		
Regular	½ cup	40
Pickled	½ cup	100
(Pathmark)	½ cup	45
(Stokely-Van Camp) pickled	½ cup	95

Food and Description	Measure or Quantity	Calories
(Town House):		
Regular	½ cup	35
Pickled	½ cup	80
Canned, dietetic, solids & liq.:		
(A&P) no salt added	½ cup	35
(Blue Boy) whole	½ cup	39
(Comstock)	½ cup	30
(Featherweight) sliced	½ cup	45
(Larsen) *Fresh-Lite*	½ cup	40
(S&W) *Nutradiet*, sliced	½ cup	35
BEET PUREE, canned (Larsen)	½ cup	45
BENEDICTINE **LIQUEUR** (Julius Wile)	1½ fl. oz.	168
BERRY BEARS, *Fruit Corners,* assorted or fruit punch	.9-oz. pkg.	100
BERRY CITRUS DRINK (Five Alive), chilled or *frozen	6 fl. oz.	88
BERRY DRINK:		
Canned, *Ssips* (Johanna Farms)	8.45-fl. oz. container	130
*Mix, dietetic, *Crystal Light*	8 fl. oz.	3
BIGG MIXX, cereal (Kellogg's):		
Plain	½ cup (1 oz.)	110
With raisins	½ cup (1.3 oz.)	140
BIG MAC (See *McDONALD'S*)		
BISCUIT DOUGH (Pillsbury):		
Baking powder, *1869 Brand*	1 biscuit	100
Buttermilk:		
Regular	1 biscuit	50
Ballard, Oven Ready	1 biscuit	50
Extra rich, *Hungry Jack*	1 biscuit	50
Fluffy, *Hungry Jack*	1 biscuit	90
Butter Tastin', 1869 Brand	1 biscuit	100
Flaky, *Hungry Jack,* regular	1 biscuit	80
Oven Ready, Ballard	1 biscuit	50
BITTERS (Angostura)	1 tsp.	14
BLACKBERRY, fresh, hulled	1 cup	84
BLACKBERRY JELLY:		
Sweetened (Home Brands)	1 T.	14
Dietetic:		
(Diet Delight)	1 T.	12
(Featherweight)	1 T.	16
BLACKBERRY LIQUEUR (Bols)	1 fl. oz.	95
BLACKBERRY PRESERVE OR JAM:		
Sweetened (Smucker's)	1 T.	53

Food and Description	Measure or Quantity	Calories
Dietetic:		
(Estee; Louis Sherry)	1 T.	6
(Featherweight)	1 T.	16
(S&W) *Nutradiet*	1 T.	12
BLACKBERRY WINE (Mogen David)	3 fl. oz.	135
BLACK-EYED PEAS:		
Canned:		
(Allen's)	½ cup	100
(Goya)	½ cup	105
(Green Giant)	½ cup	90
(Trappey's) any style	½ cup	90
(Town House)	½ cup	105
Frozen:		
(Bel-Air)	3.3 oz.	130
(Birds Eye)	⅓ pkg.	133
(Frosty Acres)	3.3 oz.	130
(McKenzie; Seabrook Farms)	⅓ pkg.	130
(Southland)	⅕ of 16-oz. pkg.	130
BLINTZ, frozen:		
(Empire Kosher):		
Apple	2½ oz.	100
Blueberry & cheese	2½ oz.	110
Potato	2½ oz.	130
(King Kold) cheese	2½ oz.	113
(King Kold) no salt added	2½ oz.	96
BLOODY MARY MIX:		
Dry (Bar-Tender's)	1 serving	26
Liquid:		
(Holland House) *Smooth 'N Spicy*	6 fl. oz.	18
(Libby's)	6 fl. oz.	40
(Sacramento)	5½-fl.-oz. can	39
Tabasco	6 fl. oz.	56
BLUEBERRY, fresh, whole	½ cup	45
BLUEBERRY PIE (See PIE, Blueberry)		
BLUEBERRY PRESERVE OR JAM:		
Sweetened:		
(Empress)	1 T.	52
(Home Brands)	1 T.	52
(Smucker's)	1 T.	54
Dietetic (Louis Sherry)	1 T.	6
BLUEFISH, broiled	3½" × 3" × ½" piece	199
BODY BUDDIES, cereal (General Mills), natural fruit flavor	⅜ cup	110

Food and Description	Measure or Quantity	Calories
BOLOGNA:		
(Boar's Head):		
Beef	1 oz.	74
Ham	1 oz.	40
Low Salt	1 oz.	80
(Butterball) turkey	1 oz.	70
(Eckrich):		
Beef:		
Regular, garlic	1 oz.	90
Thick slice	1½-oz. slice	140
German brand	1-oz. slice	80
Meat, regular	1-oz. slice	90
(Hebrew National) beef	1 oz.	90
(Hormel):		
Beef	1-oz. slice	85
Meat	1-oz. slice	90
(Louis Rich) turkey, mild	1 oz.	59
(Ohse):		
Regular	1 oz.	85
15% chicken	1 oz.	90
(Oscar Mayer):		
Beef	.5-oz. slice	48
Beef	1-oz. slice	90
Beef Lebanon	.8-oz. slice	47
Garlic beef	1-oz. slice	90
Meat	1-oz. slice	90
(Smok-A-Roma):		
Beef	1-oz. slice	90
Garlic	1-oz. slice	70
Meat:		
Regular or 15% chicken	1-oz. slice	90
Thick-sliced	1 slice	180
Turkey	1-oz. slice	60
(Swift) *Light & Lean*	1-oz. slice	95
BOLOGNA & CHEESE:		
(Eckrich)	.7-oz. slice	90
(Oscar Mayer)	.8-oz. slice	74
BONITO, canned (Star-Kist):		
Chunk	6½-oz. can	605
Solid	7-oz. can	650
BOO*BERRY, cereal (General Mills)	1 cup	110
BORSCHT, canned:		
Regular:		
(Gold's)	8-oz. serving	100
(Manischewitz) with beets	8-oz. serving	80
(Mother's) old fashioned	8-oz. serving	90
(Pepperidge Farm)	5.3-oz. serving	89

Food and Description	Measure or Quantity	Calories
(Rokeach)	8-oz. serving	96
Dietetic or low calorie:		
(Gold's)	8-oz. serving	20
(Manischewitz)	8-oz. serving	20
(Mother's):		
Artificially sweetened	8-oz. serving	29
Unsalted	8-oz. serving	107
(Rokeach):		
Diet	8-oz. serving	29
Unsalted	8-oz. serving	103
BOSCO (See SYRUP)		
BOUILLON (See specific flavor)		
BOURBON (See DISTILLED LIQUOR)		
BOYSENBERRY JELLY:		
Sweetened (Home Brands)	1 T.	15
Dietetic (S&W) *Nutradiet*, red label	1 T.	12
BOYSENBERRY JUICE, canned		
(Smucker's)	8 fl. oz.	120
BRAN:		
Crude	1 oz.	60
Miller's (Elam's)	1 oz.	87
BRAN BREAKFAST CEREAL:		
(Kellogg's):		
All Bran or *Bran Buds*	⅓ cup	70
Cracklin' Oat Bran	½ cup	110
Fruitful Bran	⅔ cup	110
Oat bran, *Common Sense,* with raisins	½ cup	120
(Loma Linda)	1 oz.	90
(Malt-O-Meal) raisin	⅜ cup	129
(Nabisco)	½ cup	70
(Post) flakes	⅔ cup	88
(Ralston Purina):		
Bran Chex	⅔ cup	90
Oat	1 cup	130
(Safeway):		
40% bran flakes	⅔ cup	90
Raisin	¾ cup	110
BRANDY (See DISTILLED LIQUOR)		
BRANDY, FLAVORED		
(Mr. Boston):		
Apricot	1 fl. oz.	94
Blackberry	1 fl. oz.	92
Cherry	1 fl. oz.	87
Ginger	1 fl. oz.	72

Food and Description	Measure or Quantity	Calories
Peach	1 fl. oz.	94
BRAUNSCHWEIGER:		
(Eckrich) chub	1 oz.	70
(Oscar Mayer) chub	1 oz.	94
(Swift) 8-oz. chub	1 oz.	109
BRAZIL NUT:		
Shelled	4 nuts	114
Roasted (Fisher) salted	1 oz.	193
BREAD, REGULAR:		
Apple cinnamon (Pritikin)	1-oz. slice	80
Autumn grain, *Merita*	1-oz. slice	75
Barbecue, *Millbrook*	1.23-oz. slice	100
Black (Mrs. Wright's)	1 slice	60
Boston brown:		
Home recipe	3" × ¾" slice	101
Canned (B&M) plain or raisin	½" slice (1.6 oz.)	80
Bran (Roman Meal):		
5 Bran	1-oz. slice	65
Oat, light	.8-oz. slice	42
Rice, honey	1-oz. slice	71
Bran'nola (Arnold)	1.3-oz. slice	90
Butter & egg (Mrs. Wright's)	1 slice	70
Buttermilk:		
Butternut or Holsum	1-oz. slice	80
Sweetheart	1-oz. slice	70
Cinnamon (Pepperidge Farm)	.9-oz. slice	90
Cracked wheat:		
(Pepperidge Farm)	1 slice	70
(Roman Meal)	1-oz. slice	67
Crispbread, *Wasa:*		
Rye, lite	.3-oz. slice	30
Sesame	.5-oz. slice	50
Date-nut roll (Dromedary)	1-oz. slice	80
Egg, *Millbrook*	1-oz. slice	70
Flatbread, *Ideal:*		
Bran	.2-oz. slice	19
Extra thin	1-oz. slice	12
Whole grain	.2-oz. slice	19
French:		
Eddy's, regular or sour	1-oz. slice	70
Francisco (Arnold)	1-oz. slice	70
(Mrs. Wright's) unsliced	.7-oz. slice	60
(Pepperidge Farm) twin	1 oz.	80
Garlic (Arnold)	1-oz. slice	80
Granola bran (Mrs. Wright's) *Grainbelt*	1 slice	140
Hi-Fibre (Monk's)	1-oz. slice	50

Food and Description	Measure or Quantity	Calories
Hillbilly, Holsum	1-oz. slice	70
Hollywood, dark	1-oz. slice	70
Honey bran (Pepperidge Farm)	1-oz. slice	90
Honey & molasses graham (Mrs. Wright's) *Grainbelt*	1 slice	100
Honey wheat berry (Arnold)	1.1-oz. slice	80
Hunters Grain, *Country Farms*	1.5-oz. slice	120
Italian (Arnold) *Francisco*	1 slice	70
Low sodium, *Butternut*	1-oz. slice	80
Multi-grain:		
(Arnold) *Milk & Honey*	1-oz. slice	70
Country Farms	1-oz. slice	80
(Pritikin)	1-oz. slice	70
(Weight Watchers)	.74-oz. slice	40
Natural grains (Arnold)	.8-oz. slice	60
Oat:		
(Arnold) *Milk & Honey*	1-oz. slice	80
(Weight Watchers)	.74-oz. slice	39
Oatmeal (Pepperidge Farm) light	1 slice	45
Olympic Meal, *Holsum*	1-oz. slice	70
Onion dill (Pritikin)	1-oz. slice	70
Pita (See *Sahara,* Thomas')		
Potato (Mrs. Wright's)	1 slice	80
Protein (Thomas')	.7-oz. slice	46
Pumpernickel:		
(Arnold)	1-oz. slice	80
(Levy's)	1.1-oz. slice	80
(Pepperidge Farm):		
Regular	1 slice	80
Party	.2-oz. slice	15
Raisin:		
(Arnold) tea	.9-oz. slice	70
(Monk's) & cinnamon	1-oz. slice	70
(Pepperidge Farm)	1 slice	90
(Pritikin)	1-oz. slice	70
(Sun-Maid)	1-oz. slice	80
(Weight Watchers)	.8-oz. slice	49
Rye:		
(Arnold) Jewish	1.1-oz. slice	80
(Levy's) real	1.1-oz. slice	80
(Mrs. Wright's):		
Regular	1 slice	60
Dill, *Grainbelt*	1 slice	100
Swedish	1-oz. slice	80
(Pepperidge Farm) family	1.1-oz. slice	80
(Pritikin)	1-oz. slice	70

Food and Description	Measure or Quantity	Calories
(Weight Watchers)	.74-oz. slice	39
(Wonder)	1-oz. slice	70
Sahara (Thomas') wheat or white	1-oz. piece	80
Sandwich (Roman Meal)	.8-oz. slice	56
Sesame seed (Mrs. Wright's)	1 slice	70
7 Grain (Roman Meal) light	.8-oz. slice	40
Sourdough, *Di Carlo*	1-oz. slice	70
Sunflower & bran (Monk's)	1-oz. slice	70
Texas toastin' (Mrs. Wright's)	1 slice	130
Vienna (Pepperidge Farm) light style	1 slice	45
Wheat (see also Cracked Wheat or Whole Wheat):		
America's Own, cottage (Arnold):	1-oz. slice	70
Bran'nola	1.3-oz. slice	80
Less or *Liteway*	.8-oz. slice	40
Fresh Horizons	1-oz. slice	50
Fresh & Natural	1-oz. slice	70
Home Pride	1-oz. slice	70
(Pepperidge Farm) family	1 slice	70
(Roman Meal)	.8-oz. slice	40
(Weight Watchers)	.74-oz. slice	40
Wheatberry, *Home Pride*, honey	1-oz. slice	70
White:		
America's Own, cottage (Arnold):	1-oz. slice	70
Brick Oven	.8-oz. slice	60
Country	1.3-oz. slice	100
Less	.8-oz. slice	40
Milk & Honey	1-oz. slice	80
Home Pride	1-oz. slice	72
(Monk's)	1-oz. slice	60
(Pepperidge Farm):		
Regular	1 slice	70
Toasting	1 slice	90
(Wonder) regular	1-oz. slice	70
Wholegrain (Roman Meal)	1-oz. slice	63
Whole wheat:		
(Arnold) *Stone Ground*	.8-oz. slice	50
(Monk's)	1-oz. slice	70
(Pepperidge Farm) thin slice	1 slice	60
(Roman Meal)	1-oz. slice	67
BREAD CRUMBS:		
(Contadina) seasoned	½ cup	211
(4C) any type	1 T.	35
(Pepperidge Farm)	1 oz.	110

Food and Description	Measure or Quantity	Calories
*BREAD DOUGH:		
Frozen:		
(Pepperidge Farm):		
Country rye or white	¹⁄₁₀ loaf	80
Stone ground wheat	¹⁄₁₀ loaf	75
(Rich's):		
French	¹⁄₂₀ loaf	59
Italian	¹⁄₂₀ loaf	60
Refrigerated (Pillsbury):		
French	1" slice	60
Wheat or white	1" slice	80
*BREAD MIX:		
Home Hearth:		
French	³⁄₈" slice	85
Rye or white	³⁄₈" slice	75
(Pillsbury):		
Banana	¹⁄₁₂ loaf	170
Cherry nut	¹⁄₁₂ loaf	180
BREAD PUDDING, with raisins, home recipe	½ cup	248
BREAD STICK (Stella D'oro):		
Plain or onion	1 piece	40
Sesame	1 piece	50
*BREAD STICK DOUGH		
(Pillsbury)	1 piece	100
BREAKFAST DRINK:		
*(Lucerne)	1 envelope	130
*(Pillsbury):		
Chocolate or strawberry	1 pouch	290
Vanilla	1 pouch	300
BRITOS, frozen (Patio):		
Beef & bean, chicken, spicy or green chili	3.6-oz. serving	250
Nacho beef	3.6-oz. serving	270
BROCCOLI:		
Boiled, with stalk	1 stalk (6.3 oz.)	47
Boiled, ½" pieces	½ cup	20
Frozen:		
(A&P) spears	3.3 oz.	25
(Bel-Air):		
Chopped, cuts or spears	3.3 oz.	25
Cuts in cheese sauce	3.3 oz.	45
(Birds Eye):		
In cheese sauce	5 oz.	132
Chopped, cuts or florets	⅓ pkg.	26
(Freezer Queen) in cheese sauce	4½ oz.	48
(Frosty Acres)	3.3 oz.	25

Food and Description	Measure or Quantity	Calories
(Green Giant):		
Cuts:		
In cream sauce:		
Regular	⅓ of 10-oz. pkg.	50
One Serving	5-oz. pkg.	70
Harvest Fresh	3 oz.	16
Polybag	½ cup	12
Spears:		
In butter sauce, regular	⅓ of 10-oz. pkg.	40
Harvest Fresh	3 oz.	19
(Larsen)	3.3 oz.	25
(Seabrook Farms) chopped or spears	⅓ of 10-oz. pkg.	30
(Stouffer's) in cheese sauce	½ of 9-oz. pkg.	130
BROTH & SEASONING:		
(George Washington)	1 packet	5
Maggi	1 T.	22
BRUNSWICK STEW, canned		
(Hormel) *Short Orders*	7½-oz. can	220
BRUSSELS SPROUT:		
Boiled	334 sprouts	28
Frozen:		
(A&P)	3.3 oz.	35
(Bel-Air)	3.3 oz.	35
(Birds Eye):		
Regular	⅓ pkg.	37
Baby, with cheese sauce	4½ oz.	128
(Frosty Acres)	3.3 oz.	35
(Green Giant):		
In butter sauce	3.3 oz.	40
Polybag	½ cup	25
BUCKWHEAT, cracked (Pocono)	1 oz.	104
*BUC*WHEATS,* cereal (General Mills)	1 oz. (⅜ cup)	110
BULGUR, canned, seasoned	4 oz.	206
BURGER KING:		
Apple pie	1 serving	311
Bagel:		
Plain	1 bagel	92
With cream cheese	1 bagel	370
Breakfast bagel sandwich:		
Plain	1 sandwich	407
Ham	1 sandwich	438
Sausage	1 sandwich	626
Breakfast Croissan'wich:		
Bacon	1 serving	355
Ham	1 serving	351
Sausage	1 serving	534

Food and Description	Measure or Quantity	Calories
Cheeseburger:		
Regular	1 serving	318
Double:		
Plain	1 serving	483
With bacon	1 serving	515
Condiments:		
Ketchup	1 serving on burger	11
Mustard	1 serving on burger	2
Pickles	1 serving on burger	0
Cherry pie	1 serving	360
Chicken sandwich:		
Regular	1 serving	685
BK Broiler	1 serving	267
Broiled without dressing	1 serving	140
Chicken Tenders	1 piece	39
Coffee, regular	1 serving	2
Danish	1 piece	500
Egg platter, scrambled:		
Bacon	1 serving	610
Sausage	1 serving	768
Fish Tenders	1 serving	265
French fries	1 regular order	227
French toast sticks	1 serving	535
Hamburger:		
Plain	1 burger	272
Condiments:		
Ketchup	1 serving on burger	11
Mustard	1 serving on burger	2
Pickles	1 serving on burger	0
Milk:		
2% low fat	1 serving	121
Whole	1 serving	157
Mocha Pie (Weight Watchers)	1 serving	160
Onion rings	1 serving	339
Orange juice	1 serving	82
Pasta (Weight Watchers):		
Angel hair:		
With cheese	1 serving	210
Without cheese	1 serving	160
Fettucini broiled chicken	1 serving	298
Salad:		
Chef	1 salad	178
Chicken	1 salad	140
Side	1 salad	25
Salad dressing:		
Regular (Newman's Own):		
Bleu Cheese	1 serving	300

Food and Description	Measure or Quantity	Calories
Ranch	1 serving	350
Thousand Island	1 serving	290
Dietetic:		
Caesar (Weight Watchers)	1 serving	6
Italian, light (Newman's Own)	1 serving	30
Ranch, creamy (Weight Watchers)	1 serving	35
Sauce:		
Barbecue (Bull's Eye)	1 T.	22
BK Broiler sauce	1 T.	90
Dipping:		
Barbecue	1 serving	45
Burger King A.M. Express Dip	1 serving	84
Honey	1 serving	91
Ranch	1 serving	171
Sweet & sour	1 serving	45
Tartar	1 serving	174
Shakes:		
Chocolate	1 shake	374
Vanilla	1 shake	334
Soft drink:		
Sweetened:		
Pepsi-Cola	1 regular size	159
7-UP	1 regular size	144
Diet *Pepsi*	1 regular size	1
Whaler:		
Plain sandwich	1 sandwich	353
Condiments:		
Lettuce	1 serving on sandwich	1
Tartar sauce	1 serving on sandwich	134
Whopper:		
Regular:		
Plain	1 sandwich	614
With cheese	1 sandwich	706
Condiments:		
Ketchup	1 serving on sandwich	17
Lettuce	1 serving on sandwich	1
Mayonnaise	1 serving on sandwich	146
Onion	1 serving on sandwich	5

Food and Description	Measure or Quantity	Calories
Pickles	1 serving on sandwich	1
Tomato	1 serving on sandwich	6
Double:		
Plain	1 sandwich	844
With cheese	1 sandwich	935
Condiments:		
Ketchup	1 serving on sandwich	8
Lettuce	1 serving on sandwich	1
Mayonnaise	1 serving on sandwich	48
Pickles	1 serving on sandwich	0
Tomato	1 serving on sandwich	3
Yogurt, frozen (Breyer's):		
Chocolate	1 serving	132
Vanilla	1 serving	120
BURGUNDY WINE:		
(Carlo Rossi)	3 fl. oz.	69
(Gallo) hearty	3 fl. oz.	69
(Louis M. Martini)	3 fl. oz.	60
(Paul Masson)	3 fl. oz.	70
(Taylor)	3 fl. oz.	75
BURGUNDY WINE, SPARKLING:		
(Carlo Rossi)	3 fl. oz.	69
(Great Western)	3 fl. oz.	82
(Taylor)	3 fl. oz.	78
BURRITO:		
*Canned (Old El Paso)	1 burrito	299
Frozen:		
(Hormel):		
Beef	1 burrito	220
Cheese	1 burrito	250
Hot chili	1 burrito	210
(Fred's) *Little Juan:*		
Bean & cheese	5-oz. serving	331
Beef & potato	5-oz. serving	389
Chili, red	10-oz. serving	799
Red hot	5-oz. serving	433
(Old El Paso):		
Regular:		
Bean & cheese	1 piece	340
Beef & bean, mild	1 piece	330

Food and Description	Measure or Quantity	Calories
Dinner, beef & bean (Patio):	11-oz. dinner	470
Beef & bean, regular	5-oz. meal	370
Red hot	5-oz. meal	360
(Swanson) bran & beef	15¼-oz. meal	720
(Van de Kamp's) regular crispy fried	6-oz. serving	365
(Weight Watchers) beefsteak or chicken	7.6-oz. meal	310
BURRITO FILLING MIX, canned (Del Monte)	½ cup	110
BURRITO SEASONING MIX (Lawry's)	1 pkg.	132
BUTTER:		
Regular:		
(Breakstone)	1 T.	100
(Meadow Gold)	1 tsp.	35
Whipped (Land O' Lakes)	1 T.	75
BUTTER SUBSTITUTE, *Butter Buds:*		
Dry or liquid	⅛ oz. dry or 1 oz. liq.	12
Sprinkles	1 tsp.	14
BUTTERSCOTCH MORSELS (Nestlés)	1 oz.	150

Food and Description	Measure or Quantity	Calories

C

CABBAGE:

Food and Description	Measure or Quantity	Calories
Boiled, until tender, without salt, drained	1 cup	29
Canned, solids & liq.:		
(Comstock) red	½ cup	60
(Greenwood)	½ cup	60
Frozen (Stouffer's) stuffed with meat, *Lean Cuisine*	10¾-oz. meal	220
CABERNET SAUVIGNON:		
(Louis M. Martini):		
Napa Valley or Sonoma County	3 fl. oz.	61
Vineyard Selection	3 fl. oz.	67
(Paul Masson)	3 fl. oz.	70
CAFE COMFORT, 55 proof	1 fl. oz.	79
CAKE:		
Regular, non-frozen:		
Plain, home recipe, with butter, with boiled white icing	⅛ of 9" square	401
Angel food:		
Home recipe	¹⁄₁₂ of 8" cake	108
(Dolly Madison)	⅙ of 10½-oz. cake	120
Apple (Dolly Madison) dutch, *Buttercrunch*	1½-oz. piece	170
Apple spice (Entenmann's) fat & cholesterol free	1-oz. slice	80
Banana crunch (Entenmann's) fat & cholesterol free	1-oz. slice	80
Blueberry crunch (Entenmann's) fat & cholesterol free	1-oz. slice	70
Butter streusel (Dolly Madison) *Buttercrumb*	1½-oz. piece	150
Caramel, home recipe, with caramel icing	⅛ of 9" square	322
Carrot (Dolly Madison) *Lunch Cake*	3¼-oz. serving	350
Chocolate, home recipe, with chocolate icing, 2-layer	¹⁄₁₂ of 9" cake	365
Chocolate (Dolly Madison) German, *Lunch Cake*	3½-oz. piece	440

Food and Description	Measure or Quantity	Calories
Chocolate loaf (Entenmann's) fat & cholesterol free	1-oz. slice	70
Cinnamon (Dolly Madison) *Buttercrumb*	1½-oz. piece	170
Creme (Dolly Madison) *Lunch Cake*	⅞-oz. cake	90
Cinnamon (Dolly Madison) *Butter Coffee*	1.3-oz. piece	90
Fruit:		
Home recipe, dark	⅟₃₀ of 8" loaf	57
Home recipe, made with butter	⅟₃₀ of 8" loaf	58
(Holland Honey Cake) unsalted	⅟₁₄ of cake	80
Golden (Entenmann's) loaf, fat & cholesterol free	1-oz. slice	80
Hawaiian spice (Dolly Madison) *Lunch Cake*	3½-oz. pkg.	350
Honey 'n spice (Dolly Madison)	3¼-oz. serving	330
Pineapple crunch (Entenmann's) fat & cholesterol free	1-oz. slice	70
Pound, home recipe, traditional, made with butter	3½" × 3½" slice	123
Raisin date loaf (Holland Honey Cake) low sodium	⅟₁₄ of 13-oz. cake	8
Sponge, home recipe	⅟₁₂ of 10" cake	196
White, home recipe, made with butter, without icing, 2-layer	⅑ of 9" wide, 3" high cake	353
White (Dolly Madison) coconut layer	⅟₁₂ of 30-oz. cake	220
Yellow, home recipe, made with butter, without icing, 2-layer	⅟₁₉ of cake	351
Frozen:		
Black forest (Weight Watchers)	3-oz. serving	180
Boston cream (Weight Watchers)	3-oz. serving	190
Carrot:		
(Pepperidge Farm) Classic	2½ oz.	260
(Weight Watchers)	3-oz. serving	170
Cheesecake:		
(Pepperidge Farm)	4¼ oz.	300
(Rich's) Viennese	⅟₁₄ of 42-oz. cake	230
(Weight Watchers):		
Regular	3.9-oz. serving	220
Strawberry	3.9-oz. serving	180
Chocolate:		
(Pepperidge Farm):		
Classic, German	2¼ oz.	250

Food and Description	Measure or Quantity	Calories
Layer:		
Fudge stripe	1⅝ oz.	170
German	1⅝ oz.	180
Light, mousse style	2½ oz.	190
(Weight Watchers) German	2½ oz.	190
Coconut (Pepperidge Farm) layer	1⅝ oz.	180
Devil's food (Pepperidge Farm) layer	⅒ of 17-oz. cake	180
Golden (Pepperidge Farm) layer	⅒ of 17-oz. cake	180
Lemon (Pepperidge Farm)	2¾ oz.	170
Pound (Pepperidge Farm) cholesterol free	1 oz.	110
Strawberry cream (Pepperidge Farm)	1/12 of 12-oz. cake	190
Vanilla (Pepperidge Farm) layer	⅒ of 17-oz. cake	190
CAKE ICING:		
Amaretto almond (Betty Crocker) *Creamy Deluxe*	1/12 can	160
Butter pecan (Betty Crocker) *Creamy Deluxe*	1/12 can	170
Caramel, home recipe	4 oz.	408
Caramel pecan (Pillsbury) *Frosting Supreme*	1/12 can	160
Cherry (Betty Crocker) *Creamy Deluxe*	1/12 can	160
Chocolate:		
(Betty Crocker) *Creamy Deluxe:*		
Regular, with candy-coated chocolate chips, with dinosaurs, milk or sour cream	1/12 can	160
Chips	1/12 can	152
(Duncan Hines):		
Fudge, dark dutch	1/12 can	149
Milk	1/12 can	151
(Mrs. Wright's) fudge creamy	1/12 can	170
(Pillsbury) *Frosting Supreme,* fudge, nut or milk	1/12 can	150
Coconut almond (Pillsbury) *Frosting Supreme*	1/12 can	150
Cream cheese:		
(Betty Crocker) *Creamy Deluxe*	1/12 can	160
(Duncan Hines)	1/12 can	152
(Pillsbury) *Frosting Supreme*	1/12 can	160
Double dutch (Pillsbury) *Frosting Supreme*	1/12 can	140
Lemon (Pillsbury) *Frosting Supreme*	1/12 can	160

Food and Description	Measure or Quantity	Calories
Polka dot (Duncan Hines) pink vanilla	¹⁄₁₂ can	154
Rainbow chip (Betty Crocker) *Creamy Deluxe*	¹⁄₁₂ can	170
Rocky road (Betty Crocker) *Creamy Deluxe*	¹⁄₁₂ can	150
Strawberry (Pillsbury) *Frosting Supreme*	¹⁄₁₂ can	160
Vanilla:		
(Betty Crocker) *Creamy Deluxe*	¹⁄₁₂ can	160
(Duncan Hines)	¹⁄₁₂ can	151
(Pillsbury) *Frosting Supreme,* regular or sour cream	¹⁄₁₂ can	160
White:		
Home recipe, boiled	4 oz.	358
Home recipe, uncooked	4 oz.	426
(Betty Crocker) *Creamy Deluxe*	¹⁄₁₂ can	160
(Mrs. Wright's)	½ can	160
*CAKE ICING MIX:		
Regular:		
Chocolate:		
Home recipe, fudge	½ cup	586
(Betty Crocker) creamy:		
Fudge	¹⁄₁₂ pkg.	180
Milk	¹⁄₁₂ pkg.	170
(Pillsbury) *Frost It Hot*	⅛ pkg.	50
Coconut almond (Pillsbury)	¹⁄₁₂ pkg.	160
Coconut pecan:		
(Betty Crocker) creamy	¹⁄₁₂ pkg.	150
(Pillsbury)	¹⁄₁₂ pkg.	150
Lemon (Betty Crocker) creamy	¹⁄₁₂ pkg.	180
Vanilla (Betty Crocker) creamy	¹⁄₁₂ pkg.	170
White:		
(Betty Crocker) fluffy	¹⁄₁₂ pkg.	70
(Betty Crocker) sour cream, creamy	¹⁄₁₂ pkg.	170
(Pillsbury) fluffy:		
Regular	¹⁄₁₂ pkg.	60
Frost It Hot	⅛ pkg.	50
Dietetic:		
(Estee)	1½ tsp.	50
(Pritikin) *Frostlite*	¹⁄₁₂ pkg.	25
CAKE OR COOKIE ICING		
(Pillsbury):		
All flavors except chocolate	1 T.	70
Chocolate	1 T.	60

Food and Description	Measure or Quantity	Calories
CAKE MEAL (Manischewitz)	½ cup	286
CAKE MIX:		
Regular:		
Angel Food:		
(Betty Crocker):		
Confetti, lemon custard or white	¹⁄₁₂ pkg.	150
Traditional	¹⁄₁₂ pkg.	130
(Duncan Hines)	¹⁄₁₂ pkg.	131
(Mrs. Wright's) deluxe	¹⁄₁₂ of cake	130
*Apple streusel (Betty Crocker) *MicroRave*:		
Regular	⅙ of cake	240
No cholesterol recipe	⅙ of cake	210
*Banana (Pillsbury) *Pillsbury Plus*	¹⁄₁₂ of cake	250
*Boston cream (Pillsbury) *Bundt*	¹⁄₁₆ of cake	270
*Butter (Pillsbury) *Pillsbury Plus*	¹⁄₁₂ of cake	260
*Butter brickle (Betty Crocker) *Supermoist*:		
Regular	¹⁄₁₂ of cake	250
No cholesterol recipe	¹⁄₁₂ of cake	220
*Butter pecan (Betty Crocker) *Supermoist*	¹⁄₁₂ of cake	250
*Carrot (Betty Crocker) *Supermoist*:		
Regular	¹⁄₁₂ of cake	250
No cholesterol recipe	¹⁄₁₂ of cake	220
*Carrot'n spice (Pillsbury) *Pillsbury Plus*	¹⁄₁₂ of cake	260
*Cheesecake:		
(Jell-O)	⅛ of 8" cake	283
(Royal) No Bake:		
Lite	⅛ of cake	210
Real	⅛ of cake	280
*Cherry chip (Betty Crocker) *Supermoist*	¹⁄₁₂ of cake	190
Chocolate:		
(Betty Crocker):		
*MicroRave:		
Fudge, with vanilla frosting	⅙ of cake	310
German, with coconut pecan frosting	⅙ of cake	320
*Pudding	⅙ of cake	230
*Supermoist:		
Chip:		
Regular	¹⁄₁₂ of cake	280

Food and Description	Measure or Quantity	Calories
No cholesterol recipe	1/12 of cake	220
Chocolate chip	1/12 of cake	260
Fudge	1/12 of cake	260
Sour cream:		
Regular	1/12 of cake	260
No cholesterol recipe	1/12 of cake	220
(Duncan Hines) fudge	1/12 pkg.	187
*(Pillsbury):		
Bundt, tunnel of fudge	1/16 of cake	260
Microwave:		
Plain	1/8 of cake	210
With chocolate frosting	1/8 of cake	300
Pillsbury Plus		
Chocolate Chip	1/12 of cake	270
Dark	1/12 of cake	250
German	1/12 of cake	250
*Cinnamon (Pillsbury) *Streusel Swirl*, microwave	1/8 of cake	240
*Cinnamon pecan streusel (Betty Crocker) *MicroRave:*		
Regular	1/6 of cake	290
No cholesterol recipe	1/6 of cake	240
Coffee cake:		
*(Aunt Jemima)	1/8 of cake	170
*(Pillsbury) Apple cinnamon	1/8 of cake	240
Devil's food:		
*(Betty Crocker):		
MicroRave, with chocolate frosting:		
Regular	1/6 of cake	310
No cholesterol recipe	1/6 of cake	240
Supermoist:		
Regular	1/12 of cake	260
No cholesterol recipe	1/12 of cake	220
(Duncan Hines) deluxe	1/12 pkg.	189
(Mrs. Wright's) deluxe	1/12 of cake	190
*(Pillsbury) *Pillsbury Plus*	1/12 of cake	270
Fudge (See Chocolate)		
Golden (Duncan Hines) butter recipe	1/12 pkg.	188
Lemon:		
(Betty Crocker) *Supermoist*	1/12 of cake	260
*(Pillsbury):		
Bundt, tunnel of	1/16 of cake	270
Streusel Swirl	1/16 of cake	270
*Lemon blueberry (Pillsbury) *Bundt*	1/16 of cake	200

Food and Description	Measure or Quantity	Calories
*Marble (Betty Crocker)		
Supermoist:		
Regular	¹⁄₁₂ of cake	250
No cholesterol recipe	¹⁄₁₂ of cake	210
*Pineapple creme (Pillsbury)		
Bundt	¹⁄₁₆ of cake	260
Pound:		
*(Betty Crocker) golden	¹⁄₁₂ of cake	200
*(Dromedary)	½" slice	150
*Rainbow chip (Betty Crocker)		
Supermoist	¹⁄₁₂ of cake	250
*Spice (Betty Crocker)		
Supermoist:		
Regular	¹⁄₁₂ of cake	260
No cholesterol recipe	¹⁄₁₂ of cake	220
*Strawberry, (Pillsbury) *Pillsbury Plus*	¹⁄₁₂ of cake	260
*Upside down (Betty Crocker) pineapple:		
Regular	¹⁄₉ of cake	250
No cholesterol recipe	¹⁄₉ of cake	240
*Vanilla (Betty Crocker) golden:		
MicroRave	¹⁄₆ of cake	320
Supermoist, regular	¹⁄₁₂ of cake	280
White:		
*(Betty Crocker) *Supermoist*:		
Regular	¹⁄₁₂ of cake	240
Sour cream	¹⁄₁₂ of cake	180
(Duncan Hines) deluxe	¹⁄₁₂ pkg.	188
*(Mrs. Wright's) deluxe	¹⁄₁₂ of cake	180
Yellow:		
*(Betty Crocker):		
MicroRave, with chocolate frosting:		
Regular	¹⁄₆ of cake	300
No cholesterol recipe	¹⁄₆ of cake	230
Supermoist:		
Regular	¹⁄₁₂ of cake	260
No cholesterol recipe	¹⁄₁₂ of cake	220
(Duncan Hines) deluxe	¹⁄₁₂ pkg.	188
*(Mrs. Wright) deluxe	¹⁄₁₂ of cake	190
*(Pillsbury):		
*Microwave, plain	¹⁄₈ of cake	220
Pillsbury Plus	¹⁄₁₂ of cake	260
*Dietetic:		
(Estee) any flavor	¹⁄₁₀ of cake	100
(Pritikin) *Batterlite,* unfrosted	¹⁄₁₀ of cake	90

Food and Description	Measure or Quantity	Calories
CAMPARI, 45 proof	1 fl. oz.	66
CANDY, REGULAR:		
Almond, Jordan (Banner)	1¼-oz. box	154
Almond Joy (Hershey's)	1.76-oz. bar	250
Apricot Delight (Sahadi)	1 oz.	100
Baby Ruth	2-oz. piece	260
Bar None (Hershey's)	1½ oz.	240
Bit-O-Honey (Nestlé)	1 oz.	120
Bonkers! any flavor	1 piece	20
Breath Savers (Life Savers)	1 piece	8
Butterfinger	2-oz. bar	260
Butternut (Hollywood Brands)	2¼-oz. bar	310
Caramel:		
Caramel Flipper (Wayne)	1 oz.	128
Caramel Nip (Pearson)	1 piece	30
Caramello (Hershey's)	1.6-oz. bar	220
Charleston Chew	2-oz. piece	240
Cherry, chocolate-covered		
(*Welch's*) dark	1 piece	90
Chocolate bar:		
Alpine white (Nestlé)	1 oz.	170
Brazil nut (Cadbury's)	2 oz.	310
Caramello (Cadbury's)	2 oz.	280
Crunch (Nestlé)	1¹⁄₁₆-oz. bar	160
Hazelnut (Cadbury's)	2 oz.	310
Milk:		
(Cadbury's)	2 oz.	300
(Hershey's)	1.55-oz. bar	240
(Nestlé)	.35-oz. bar	53
(Nestlé)	1¹⁄₁₆-oz. bar	159
Special Dark (Hershey's)	1.45-oz. bar	220
Chocolate bar with almonds:		
(Cadbury's)	2 oz.	310
(Hershey's):		
Regular	1.45-oz. bar	230
Golden Almond	3.2-oz. bar	520
(Nestlé)	1 oz.	160
Chocolate Parfait (Pearson)	1 piece	30
Chocolate, Petite (Andes)	1 piece	26
Chuckles	1 oz.	92
Chunky (Nestlé):		
Regular	1 oz.	150
Deluxe nut	1 oz.	160
Clark Bar	1.5-oz. bar	201
Coffee Nip (Pearson)	1 piece	30
Coffioca Parfait (Pearson)	1 piece	30
Creme de Menthe (Andes)	1 piece	25

Food and Description	Measure or Quantity	Calories
Crispy Bar (Clark)	1¼-oz. bar	187
Crows (Mason)	1 piece	11
Dutch Treat Bar (Clark)	1¹⁄₁₆-oz. bar	160
Eggs (Hershey's) creme	1 oz.	136
5th Avenue (Hershey's)	2.1-oz. bar	290
Fruit bears (Flavor Tree) assorted	½ of 2.1-oz. envelope	117
Fruit circus (Flavor Tree)	½ of 2.1-oz. envelope	117
Fruit roll (Flavor Tree):		
Apple or cherry	¾-oz. roll	75
Strawberry	¾-oz. roll	74
Fudge (Nabisco) bar	1 piece	85
Goobers (Nestlé)	1 oz.	160
Good Stuff (Nab)	1.8-oz. piece	250
Halvah (Sahadi) original and marble	1 oz.	150
Hard (Jolly Rancher):		
All flavors except butterscotch	1 piece	23
Butterscotch	1 piece	25
Hollywood	1½-oz. bar	185
Jelly bean (*Chuckles*)	.5 oz.	55
Jelly rings (*Chuckles*)	1 piece	37
Jujubes (*Chuckles*)	.5 oz.	55
Ju Jus:		
Assorted	1 piece	7
Coins or raspberries	1 piece	15
Kisses (Hershey's)	1 piece	24
Kit Kat	1.6-oz. bar	250
Krackel Bar	1.55-oz. bar	230
Licorice:		
(Switzer) bars, bites or stix:		
Black	1 oz.	94
Cherry or strawberry	1 oz.	98
Chocolate	1 oz.	97
Twist:		
Black (American Licorice Co.)	1 piece	27
Black (Curtiss)	1 piece	27
Red (American Licorice Co.)	1 piece	33
Life Savers	1 piece	10
Lollipops (Life Savers)	1 pop	45
Mallo Cup (Boyer)	⁹⁄₁₆-oz. piece	54
Malted milk balls (Brach's)	1 piece	9
Mars Bar (M&M/Mars)	1.7-oz. bar	240
Marshmallow (Campfire)	1 oz.	111
Mary Jane (Miller):		
Small size	1.4 oz.	19

Food and Description	Measure or Quantity	Calories
Large size	1½-oz. bar	110
Milk Duds (Clark)	¾-oz. box	89
Milk Shake (Hollywood Brands)	2.4-oz. bar	300
Milky Way (M&M/Mars)	2.24-oz. bar	290
Mint or peppermint:		
After dinner (Richardson):		
Jelly center	1 oz.	104
Regular	1 oz.	109
Canada Mint (Necco)	1 oz.	12
Chocolate-covered (Richardson)	1 oz.	106
Junior mint pattie (Nabisco)	1 piece	10
Mint Parfait (Andes)	1 piece	27
Peppermint Pattie (Nabisco)	1 piece	55
York, pattie (Hershey's)	1.5-oz.	180
M&M's:		
Peanut	1.83-oz. pkg.	270
Plain	1.69-oz. pkg.	240
Mounds (Hershey's)	1.9-oz. serving	260
Mr. Goodbar (Hershey's)	1.75-oz. bar	290
Munch Bar (M&M/Mars)	1.42-oz. bar	220
My Buddy (Tom's)	1.8-oz. piece	250
Naturally Nut & Fruit Bar (Planters) almond/apricot	1 oz.	140
Necco Wafers, assorted	2.02-oz. roll	227
Nibs (Y&S)	1 oz.	100
Oh Henry! (Nestlé)	1 oz.	140
$100,000 Bar (Nestlé)	1.5-oz. bar	200
Orange slices (*Chuckles*)	1 oz.	110
Park Avenue (Tom's)	1.8-oz. bar	230
Payday (Hollywood Brands) regular	1.9-oz. bar	250
Peanut, chocolate-covered:		
(Curtiss)	1 piece	5
(Nabisco)	1 piece	11
Peanut bar (Planters)	1.6 oz.	240
Peanut butter cookie bar (M&M/Mars)	1⅜-oz. serving	261
Peanut butter cup:		
(Boyer)	1.5-oz. pkg.	148
(Reese's)	.9-oz. cup	140
Peanut Butter Pals (Tom's)	1.3-oz. serving	200
Peanut crunch bar (Sahadi)	⅜-oz. bar	110
Peanut Parfait (Andes)	1 piece	28
Peanut Plank (Tom's)	1.7-oz. piece	230
Peanut Roll (Tom's)	1.75-oz. piece	230
Powerhouse (Hershey's)	2 oz.	260
Raisin, chocolate-covered:		
(Nabisco)	1 piece	5

Food and Description	Measure or Quantity	Calories
Raisinets (Nestlé)	1 oz.	120
Reese's Pieces (Hershey's)	1 piece	32
Reggie Bar	2-oz. bar	290
Rolo (Hershey's)	1 piece	34
Royals, mint chocolate (M&M/ Mars)	1.52-oz. pkg.	212
Sesame Crunch (Sahadi)	⅜-oz. bar	110
Skor (Hershey's)	1.4-oz. bar	220
Sky Bar (Necco)	1.5-oz. bar	198
Snickers	2-oz. bar	290
Solitaires (Hershey's)	½ of 3.2-oz. pkg.	260
Spearmint leaves (*Chuckles*)	1 oz.	110
Starburst (M&M/Mars)	1-oz. serving	120
Sugar Babies (Nabisco)	1.6-oz. pkg.	180
Sugar Daddy (Nabisco) caramel sucker	1.4-oz. pop	150
Sugar Mama (Nabisco)	⅜-oz. pop	90
Summit (M&M/Mars)	1 bar	115
Symphony (Hershey's)	1.4-oz. serving	220
Taffy, salt water (Brach's)	1 piece	31
3 Musketeers	.8-oz. bar	99
3 Musketeers	2.1-oz. bar	260
Ting-A-Ling (Andes)	1 piece	24
Tootsie Roll:		
Chocolate	.23-oz. midgee	26
Chocolate	1/16-oz. bar	72
Chocolate	1-oz. bar	115
Flavored	.6-oz. square	19
Pop, all flavors	.49-oz. pop	55
Pop drop, all flavors	4.7-gram piece	19
Twix (M&M/Mars)	1¾-oz. serving	246
Twizzlers	1 oz.	100
Whatchamacallit (Hershey's)	1.8-oz. bar	260
Wispa (Hershey's)	1 oz.	150
World Series Bar	1 oz.	128
Y & S Bites	1 oz.	100
Zagnut Bar (Clark)	.7-oz. bar	85
Zero (Hollywood Brands)	2-oz. bar	210
CANDY, DIETETIC:		
Caramel (Estee) chocolate or vanilla	1 piece	30
Carob bar, *Joan's Natural:*		
Coconut	3-oz. bar	516
Fruit & nut	3-oz. bar	559
Honey bran	3-oz. bar	487
Peanut	3-oz. bar	521

Food and Description	Measure or Quantity	Calories
Chocolate or chocolate-flavored bar:		
(Estee):		
Coconut, fruit & nut or milk	.2-oz. square	30
Crunch	.2-oz. square	22
(Louis Sherry) coffee or orange-flavored	.2-oz. square	22
Estee-ets, with peanuts (Estee)	1 piece	7
Gum drops (Estee) any flavor	1 piece	6
Gummy Bears (Estee)	1 piece	7
Hard candy:		
(Estee) assorted fruit	1 piece	12
(Louis Sherry)	1 piece	12
Peanut brittle (Estee)	¼ oz.	35
Peanut butter cup (Estee)	1 cup	40
Raisins, chocolate-covered (Estee)	1 piece	3
CANDY APPLE COOLER DRINK, canned (Hi-C)	6 fl. oz.	94
CANNELLONI, frozen:		
(Armour) *Dining Lite*, cheese	9-oz. dinner	310
(Celentano)	12-oz. pkg.	350
(Stouffer's) beef & pork with mornay sauce, *Lean Cuisine*	9⅝-oz. pkg.	260
CANTALOUPE, cubed	½ cup (3 oz.)	24
CAPERS (Crosse & Blackwell)	1 tsp.	2
CAP'N CRUNCH, cereal (Quaker):		
Regular	¾ cup	121
Crunchberry	¾ cup	120
Peanut butter	¾ cup	127
CAPOCOLLO (Hormel)	1 oz.	80
CARAWAY SEED (French's)	1 tsp.	8
CARL'S JR. RESTAURANT:		
Bacon	2 strips (10 grams)	50
Cake, chocolate	3.2-oz. piece	380
California Roast Beef 'n Swiss sandwich	7.2-oz. sandwich	360
Cheese:		
American	.6-oz. slice	63
Swiss	.6-oz. slice	57
Chicken sandwich:		
Charbroiler BBQ	6.3-oz. sandwich	320
Charbroiler Club	8.2-oz. sandwich	510
Cookie, chocolate chip	2¼-oz. piece	330
Danish	3.5-oz. piece	300
Eggs, scrambled	2.4-oz. serving	120
Fish sandwich, filet	7.9-oz. sandwich	550

Food and Description	Measure or Quantity	Calories
French toast dips, excluding syrup	4.7-oz. serving	480
Hamburger:		
Plain:		
Famous Star	8.1-oz. serving	590
Happy Star	3.0-oz. serving	220
Old Time Star	5.9-oz. serving	400
Super Star	10.6-oz. serving	770
Cheeseburger, *Western Bacon:*		
Regular	7½-oz. serving	630
Double	10.4-oz. serving	890
Hot cake, with margarine, excluding syrup	5.5-oz. serving	360
Milk, 2% lowfat	10 fl. oz.	175
Muffins:		
Blueberry	3.5-oz. piece	256
Bran	4-oz. piece	220
English, with margarine	2-oz. piece	180
Onion rings	3.2-oz. order	310
Orange juice, small	8 fl. oz.	94
Potato:		
Baked:		
Bacon & cheese	14.1-oz. serving	650
Broccoli & cheese	14-oz. serving	470
Cheese	14.2-oz. serving	550
Fiesta	15.2-oz. serving	550
Lite	9.8-oz. serving	250
Sour cream & chive	10.4-oz. serving	350
French fries	Regular order (6 oz.)	360
Hash brown nuggets	3-oz. serving	170
Salad dressing:		
Regular:		
Blue cheese	2-oz. serving	150
House	2-oz. serving	186
1000 Island	2-oz. serving	231
Dietetic, Italian	2-oz. serving	80
Sausage patty	1.5-oz. piece	190
Shake	1 regular size	353
Soft drink:		
Sweetened	1 regular size	243
Dietetic	1 regular size	2
Soup:		
Broccoli, cream of	1 serving	140
Chicken & noodle	1 serving	80
Clam chowder, Boston	1 serving	140
Vegetable, mixed	1 serving	70

Food and Description	Measure or Quantity	Calories
Steak sandwich, *Country Fried Sunrise Sandwich:*	7.2-oz. serving	610
Bacon	4.5-oz. serving	370
Sausage	6.1-oz. serving	500
Tea, iced	1 regular drink	2
Zucchini	4.3-oz. serving	300
CARNATION DO-IT-YOURSELF DIET PLAN	2 scoops	110
CARNATION INSTANT BREAKFAST:		
Bar:		
Chocolate chip	1 bar	200
Peanut butter crunch	1 bar	180
Packets, all flavors	1 packet	130
CARROT:		
Raw	5½" 1" piece	21
Boiled, slices	½ cup	24
Canned, regular pack, solids & liq.:		
(A&P)	½ cup	30
(Larsen) *Freshlike*	½ cup	0
(Libby's)	½ cup	20
Canned, dietetic pack, solids & liq., (S&W) *Nutradiet,* green label	½ cup	30
Frozen:		
(Bel-Air) whole, baby	3.3 oz.	40
(Birds Eye) deluxe	2.7 oz.	32
(Frosty Acres)	3.3 oz.	40
(Green Giant) cuts, in butter sauce	½ cup	80
(Larsen)	3.3 oz.	40
(Seabrook Farms)	⅓ pkg.	39
CARROT JUICE, canned (Hain)	6 fl. oz.	30
CASABA MELON	1-lb. melon	61
CASHEW BUTTER (Hain)	1 T.	95
CASHEW NUT:		
(Eagle Snacks) honey roast	1 oz.	170
(Fisher):		
Dry roasted	1 oz.	156
Honey, salted	1 oz.	150
Oil roasted	1 oz.	159
(Party Pride) dry roasted	1 oz.	170
(Planters):		
Dry roasted	1 oz.	160
Honey roasted	1 oz.	170
Oil roasted	1 oz.	170
CATFISH, frozen (Mrs. Paul's) breaded & fried, fingers	4 oz.	250

Food and Description	Measure or Quantity	Calories
CATSUP:		
Regular:		
(Heinz)	1 T.	18
(Hunt's)	1 T.	15
(Smucker's)	1 T.	24
(Town House)	1 T.	15
Dietetic or low calorie:		
(Del Monte) no salt added	1 T.	15
(Estee)	1 T.	6
(Featherweight)	1 T.	6
(Heinz) lite	1 T.	18
(Hunt's)	1 T.	20
(Weight Watchers)	1 T.	12
CAULIFLOWER:		
Raw or boiled buds	½ cup	14
Frozen:		
(A&P)	3.3 oz.	25
(Bel-Air)	3.3 oz.	25
(Birds Eye) regular	3.3 oz.	23
(Budget Gourmet) in cheddar cheese sauce	5 oz.	110
(Frosty Acres)	3.3 oz.	25
(Green Giant):		
In cheese sauce:		
Regular	⅓ of 10-oz. pkg.	50
One Serving	5½-oz. serving	80
Polybag, cuts	2 oz.	12
(Larsen)	3.3 oz.	25
CAULIFLOWER, PICKLED		
(Vlasic) sweet	1 oz.	35
CAVATELLI, frozen		
(Celentano)	⅕ of 16-oz. pkg.	250
CAVIAR:		
Pressed	1 oz.	90
Whole eggs	1 T.	42
CELERY:		
1 large outer stalk	8" × 1½" at root end	7
Diced or cut	½ cup	9
Frozen (Larsen)	3½ oz.	14
CELERY SALT (French's)	1 tsp.	12
CELERY SEED (French's)	1 tsp.	11
CEREAL (See brand name or specific type)		
CEREAL BAR (Kellogg's) *Smart Start*: *Common Sense*, oat bran with raspberry filling	1½-oz. bar	170

Food and Description	Measure or Quantity	Calories
Nutri-Grain	1½-oz. bar	180
Rice Krispies, with almonds	1-oz. bar	130
CERTS	1 piece	6
CERVELAT (Hormel) Viking	1-oz. serving	90
CHABLIS WINE:		
(Almaden) light	3 fl. oz.	42
(Carlo Rossi)	3 fl. oz.	63
(Gallo) white or pink	3 fl. oz.	60
(Louis M. Martini)	3 fl. oz.	59
(Paul Masson):		
Regular	3 fl. oz.	71
Light	3 fl. oz.	45
CHAMPAGNE:		
(Bollinger)	3 fl. oz.	72
(Great Western):		
Regular	3 fl. oz.	71
Brut	3 fl. oz.	74
Pink	3 fl. oz.	81
(Taylor) dry	3 fl. oz.	78
CHARDONNAY WINE:		
(Gallo)	3 fl. oz.	66
(Louis M. Martini)	3 fl. oz.	60
CHARLOTTE RUSSE, homemade recipe	4 oz.	324
CHEERIOS, cereal, (General Mills), regular, apple cinnamon, or honey & nut	1 oz.	110
CHEESE:		
American or cheddar:		
Cube, natural	1" cube	68
(Alpine Lace)	1 oz.	80
(Borden)	1 oz.	110
(Churny) lite, cheddar, mild	1 oz.	80
(Dorman's):		
American:		
Lo-chol	1 oz.	90
Low sodium	1 oz.	110
Cheddar, light	1 oz.	80
(Hickory Farms)	1 oz.	110
(Kraft):		
American Singles	1 oz.	90
Cheddar	1 oz.	110
Old English	1 oz.	110
(Land O' Lakes):		
Regular or with bacon	1 oz.	110
Chederella	1 oz.	100
Sharp or extra sharp	1 oz.	100

Food and Description	Measure or Quantity	Calories
Laughing Cow, natural	1 oz.	110
(Lucerne) American slices or cheddar	1 oz.	110
(Polly-O) cheddar, shredded	1 oz.	110
(Safeway)	1 oz.	110
(Sargento):		
Midget, regular or sharp	1 oz.	114
Shredded, non-dairy	1 oz.	90
(Weight Watchers) natural, low sodium	1 oz.	80
Wispride	1 oz.	115
Blue:		
(Frigo)	1 oz.	100
(Hickory Farms) domestic	1 oz.	101
(Kraft)	1 oz.	100
(Safeway) imported Danish or Treasure Cave	1 oz.	100
(Sargento) cold pack or crumbled	1 oz.	100
Bonbino, *Laughing Cow,* natural	1 oz.	103
Brick:		
(Land O' Lakes)	1 oz.	110
(Safeway) mild	1 oz.	100
(Sargento) sliced	1 oz.	105
Brie (Sargento) *Danish Danko*	1 oz.	80
Burgercheese (Sargento) *Danish Danko*	1 oz.	106
Camembert (Sargento) *Danish Danko*	1 oz.	88
Colby:		
(Alpine Lace)	1 oz.	80
(Churny) lite	1 oz.	80
(Dorman's) *Lo-Chol*	1 oz.	100
(Hickory Farms) Longhorn	1 oz.	112
(Kraft)	1 oz.	110
(Land O' Lakes)	1 oz.	110
(Lucerne) loaf or shredded	1 oz.	110
(Pauly) low sodium	1 oz.	115
(Safeway)	1 oz.	110
(Sargento) shredded or sliced	1 oz.	112
(Weight Watchers)	1 oz.	80
Cottage:		
Unflavored:		
(Bison):		
Regular	1 oz.	29
Dietetic	1 oz.	22
(Borden):		
Regular, 4% milkfat	½ cup	120

Food and Description	Measure or Quantity	Calories
Lite-Line, 1.5% milkfat	½ cup	90
(Breakstone's) smooth & creamy	1 oz.	27
(Dairylea)	1 oz.	30
(Friendship)	1 oz.	30
(Johanna Farms):		
Large or small curd	½ cup	120
No salt added	½ cup	90
(Land O' Lakes)	1 oz.	30
(Light n' Lively)	1 oz.	20
(Lucerne):		
Dry curd	¼ cup	40
Farmer curd	¼ cup	60
Low fat, regular or unsalted	¼ cup	50
(Sealtest)	1 oz.	30
(Weight Watchers) 1%	½ cup	90
Flavored (Friendship) pineapple	1 oz.	35
Cream, plain, unwhipped:		
(Alpine Lace) fat free	1 oz.	30
(Frigo)	1 oz.	100
(Kraft) *Philadelphia Brand*:		
Regular	1 oz.	100
Light	1 oz.	60
(Lucerne) plain, regular or soft	1 oz.	100
Edam:		
(Churny) *May-Bud*	1 oz.	100
(Kaukauna)	1 oz.	100
(Land O' Lakes)	1 oz.	100
Laughing Cow	1 oz.	100
(Safeway)	1 oz.	100
Farmer:		
(Churny) *May-Bud*	1 oz.	90
Dutch Garden Brand	1 oz.	100
(Hickory Farms)	1 oz.	90
(Kaukauna)	1 oz.	100
(Sargento)	1 oz.	72
Wispride	1 oz.	100
Feta (Sargento) cups	1 oz.	76
Fontina (Safeway)	1 oz.	110
Gjetost (Sargento) Norwegian	1 oz.	118
Gouda:		
(Churny) *May-Bud*, lite	1 oz.	81
(Kaukauna)	1 oz.	100
(Land O' Lakes)	1 oz.	100
(Lucerne)	1 oz.	100
Wispride	1 oz.	100
Grated (Polly-O)	1 oz.	130

Food and Description	Measure or Quantity	Calories
Gruyère, *Swiss Knight*	1 oz.	100
Havarti (Sargento):		
Creamy	1 oz.	90
Creamy, 60% mild	1 oz.	117
Hoop (Friendship) natural	1 oz.	21
Hot pepper (Sargento)	1 oz.	112
Jalapeño Jack (Land O'Lakes)	1 oz.	90
Jarlsberg (Sargento) Norwegian	1 oz.	100
Kettle Moraine (Sargento)	1 oz.	100
Limburger (Sargento) natural	1 oz.	100
Longhorn (Safeway)	1 oz.	110
Monterey Jack:		
(Churny) lite	1 oz.	80
(Kaukauna)	1 oz.	110
(Land O' Lakes)	1 oz.	110
(Lucerne)	1 oz.	105
(Sargento) midget, Longhorn, shredded or sliced	1 oz.	106
(Weight Watchers)	1 oz.	80
Mozzarella:		
(Alpine Lace) Free 'N Lean	1 oz.	40
(Kraft)	1 oz.	80
(Lucerne)	1 oz.	80
(Polly-O):		
Fior di Latte	1 oz.	80
Part skim milk	1 oz.	80
Smoked	1 oz.	85
Whole milk:		
Regular or shredded	1 oz.	90
Old fashioned, regular	1 oz.	70
(Safeway) regular or stick	1 oz.	80
(Sargento):		
Bar, rounds, shredded regular or with spices, sliced for pizzas or square	1 oz.	79
Whole milk	1 oz.	100
(Weight Watchers) shredded	1 oz.	70
Muenster:		
(Alpine Lace)	1 oz.	100
(Dorman's):		
Light	1 oz.	80
Lo-chol	1 oz.	100
Low sodium	1 oz.	110
(Hickory Farms)	1 oz.	100
(Kaukauna)	1 oz.	110
(Land O' Lakes)	1 oz.	100
(Safeway) orange rind	1 oz.	105

Food and Description	Measure or Quantity	Calories
(Sargento) red rind	1 oz.	104
Wispride	1 oz.	100
Nibblin Curds (Sargento)	1 oz.	114
Parmesan:		
(Lucerne)	1 oz.	110
(Polly-O) grated	1 oz.	130
(Progresso) grated	1 T.	23
(Sargento):		
Grated	1 T.	27
Wedge	1 oz.	110
Pizza (Sargento) shredded or sliced	1 oz.	90
Pot (Sargento) regular, French onion or garlic	1 oz.	30
Provolone:		
(Alpine Lace) *Provo-Lo*	1 oz.	70
(Dorman's) light	1 oz.	80
(Land O' Lakes)	1 oz.	100
Laughing Cow:		
Cube	⅙ oz.	12
Wedge	⅜ oz.	55
(Lucerne) sliced	1 oz.	100
(Safeway)	1 oz.	100
(Sargento) sliced	1 oz.	100
Ricotta:		
(Frigo) part skim milk	1 oz.	43
(Polly-O):		
Lite	1 oz.	40
Part skim milk	1 oz.	45
Whole milk	1 oz.	50
(Sargento):		
Part skim milk	1 oz.	39
Whole milk	1 oz.	49
Romano:		
(Polly-O) grated	1 oz.	130
(Progresso) grated	1 T.	23
(Sargento) wedge	1 oz.	110
Roquefort, natural	1 oz.	104
Samsoe (Sargento) Danish	1 oz.	79
Scamorze (Frigo)	1 oz.	79
Semisoft, *Laughing Cow:*		
Babybel	1 oz.	90
Bonbel	1 oz.	100
Slim Jack (Dorman's)	1 oz.	80
Stirred curd (Frigo)	1 oz.	110
String (Sargento)	1 oz.	90
Swiss:		
(Alpine Lace) *Swiss-Lo*	1 oz.	100

Food and Description	Measure or Quantity	Calories
(Churny) lite	1 oz.	90
(Dorman's) light	1 oz.	90
(Hickory Farms) *Light Choice*, low sodium	1 oz.	100
(Lucerne)	1 oz.	100
(Sargento) domestic or Finland, sliced	1 oz.	107
Taco (Sargento) shredded	1 oz.	105
Washed curd (Frigo)	1 oz.	110
CHEESE FONDUE, *Swiss Knight*	1 oz.	110
CHEESE FOOD:		
American or cheddar:		
(Borden) *Lite-Line*	1 oz.	50
(Fisher) *Ched-O-Mate* or *Sandwich-Mate*	1 oz.	90
Heart Beat (GFA)	⅔-oz. slice	35
(Lucerne)	1 oz.	90
(Weight Watchers) colored or white	1-oz. slice	50
Wispride:		
Regular	1 oz.	100
& port wine	1 oz.	100
Cheez-ola (Fisher)	1 oz.	90
Chef's Delight (Fisher)	1 oz.	70
Count Down (Pauly)	1 oz.	40
Cracker snack (Sargento)	1 oz.	90
Garlic & herbs, *Wispride*	1 oz.	90
Hot pepper (Lucerne)	1 oz.	90
Italian herb (Land O' Lakes)	1 oz.	90
Jalapeño (Borden) *Lite-Line*	1 oz.	50
Loaf, *Count Down* (Pauly)	1 oz.	100
Low sodium:		
(Borden) *Lite-Line*	1 oz.	70
Heart Beat (GFA)	.7-oz. slice	35
Monterey Jack (Borden) *Lite-Line*	1 oz.	50
Mun-chee (Pauly)	1 oz.	100
Neufchatel (Shedd's) Country Crock, any flavor	1 oz.	70
Onion (Land O' Lakes)	1 oz.	90
Pepperoni (Land O' Lakes)	1 oz.	90
Pimiento (Pauly)	.8-oz. slice	73
Pizza-Mate (Fisher)	1 oz.	90
Salami (Land O' Lakes)	1 oz.	90
Swiss:		
(Borden) *Lite-Line*	1 oz.	50
(Kraft) reduced fat	1 oz.	90

Food and Description	Measure or Quantity	Calories
CHEESE SPREAD:		
American or cheddar:		
(Fisher)	1 oz.	80
Laughing Cow	1 oz.	72
(Nabisco) *Easy Cheese*	1 tsp.	16
Blue, *Laughing Cow*	1 oz.	72
Cheese'n Bacon (Nabisco) *Easy Cheese*	1 tsp.	16
Golden velvet (Land O' Lakes)	1 oz.	80
Gruyère, *Laughing Cow, La Vache Que Rit,* reduced calorie	1 oz.	46
Provolone, *Laughing Cow*	1 oz.	72
Sharp (Pauly)	.8 oz.	77
Swiss, process (Pauly)	.8 oz.	76
Velveeta (Kraft)	1 oz.	80
CHENIN BLANC WINE:		
(Gallo)	3 fl. oz.	64
(Louis M. Martini)	3 fl. oz.	56
CHERRY, SWEET:		
Fresh, with stems	½ cup (2.3 oz.)	41
Canned, regular pack (Del Monte) dark, solids & liq.	½ cup	50
Canned, dietetic, solids & liq.:		
(Diet Delight) with pits, water pack	½ cup	70
(Featherweight) dark, water pack	½ cup	60
(Thank You Brand)	½ cup	61
CHERRY, CANDIED	1 oz.	96
CHERRY DRINK:		
Canned:		
(Hi-C)	6 fl. oz.	100
(Lincoln) cherry berry	6 fl. oz.	100
(Smucker's) black	8 fl. oz.	130
Squeezit (General Mills)	6¾-fl.-oz. container	110
Ssips (Johanna Farms)	8.45-fl.-oz. container	130
*Mix (Funny Face)	8 fl. oz.	88
CHERRY HEERING		
(Hiram Walker)	1 fl. oz.	80
CHERRY JELLY:		
Sweetened (Smucker's)	1 T.	54
Dietetic:		
(Dia-Mel)	1 T.	6
(Featherweight)	1 T.	16
(Smucker's)	⅜-oz. packet	4
CHERRY LIQUEUR (DeKuyper)	1 fl. oz.	75

Food and Description	Measure or Quantity	Calories
CHERRY PRESERVES OR JAM:		
Sweetened (Smucker's)	1 T.	54
Dietetic (Estee)	1 T.	6
CHESTNUT, fresh, in shell	¼ lb.	220
CHEWING GUM:		
Sweetened:		
Bazooka, bubble	1 slice	18
Beechies	1 piece	6
Beech Nut; Beeman's Big Red; Black Jack; Clove; Doublemint; Freedent; Juicy Fruit, Spearmint (Wrigley's); *Teaberry*	1 stick	10
Bubble Yum	1 piece	25
Dentyne	1 piece	4
Extra (Wrigley's)	1 piece	8
Fruit Stripe, regular	1 piece	9
Hubba Bubba (Wrigley's)	1 piece	23
Dietetic:		
Bubble Yum	1 piece	20
Care Free, regular	1 piece	8
(Clark; *Care Free*)	1 piece	7
(Estee) bubble or regular	1 piece	5
Extra (Wrigley's) cinnamon or spearmint	1 piece	8
(Featherweight) bubble or regular	1 piece	4
CHEX, cereal (Ralston Purina):		
Corn	1 cup (1 oz.)	110
Honey graham	⅔ cup	110
Rice	1⅛ cup (1 oz.)	110
Wheat	⅔ cup (1 oz.)	100
CHIANTI WINE:		
(Carlo Rossi) light	3 fl. oz.	69
(Italian Swiss Colony)	3 fl. oz.	83
(Louis M. Martini)	3 fl. oz.	90
CHICKEN:		
Broiler, cooked, meat only	3 oz.	116
Fryer, fried, meat & skin	3 oz.	212
Fryer, fried, meat only	3 oz.	178
Fryer, fried, 2½-lb. chicken (weighed with bone before cooking) will give you:		
Back	1 back	139
Breast	½ breast	160
Leg or drumstick	1 leg	87
Neck	1 neck	127

Food and Description	Measure or Quantity	Calories
Rib	1 rib	41
Thigh	1 thigh	122
Wing	1 wing	82
Fried skin	1 oz.	119
Hen & cock:		
Stewed, dark meat only	3 oz.	176
Stewed, diced	½ cup	139
Stewed, light meat only	3 oz.	153
Stewed, meat & skin	3 oz.	269
Roaster, roasted, dark or light meat, without skin	3 oz.	156
CHICKEN À LA KING:		
Home recipe	1 cup	468
Canned (Swanson)	½ of 10½-oz. can	190
Frozen:		
(Armour) *Classics Lite*	11¼-oz. meal	290
(Banquet) *Cookin' Bag*	4-oz. pkg.	110
(Kraft)	10-oz. meal	350
(Le Menu):		
Regular	10¼-oz. dinner	330
Healthy entree	8¼-oz. entree	240
(Stouffer's) with rice	9½-oz. pkg.	290
(Weight Watchers)	9-oz. pkg.	220
CHICKEN, BONED, canned:		
Regular:		
(Hormel) chunk, breast	6¾-oz. serving	350
(Swanson) chunk:		
Mixin' chicken	2½ oz.	130
White	2½ oz.	100
Low sodium (Featherweight)	2½ oz.	75
CHICKEN BOUILLON:		
Regular:		
(Herb-Ox):		
Cube	1 cube	6
Packet	1 packet	12
(Knorr)	1 cube	16
(Wyler's)	1 cube	8
Low sodium:		
(Borden) *Lite-Line*	1 tsp.	12
(Featherweight)	1 tsp.	18
CHICKEN CHUNKS, frozen		
(Country Pride):		
Regular	¼ of 12-oz. pkg.	240
Southern fried	¼ of 12-oz. pkg.	280
CHICKEN, CREAMED, frozen		
(Stouffer's)	6½ oz.	300

Food and Description	Measure or Quantity	Calories
CHICKEN DINNER OR ENTREE:		
Canned:		
*(Hormel) Top Shelf:		
Acapulco	1 serving	390
Breast of, glazed	1 serving	210
Sweet & sour	1 serving	270
(Hunt's) *Minute Gourmet Microwave Entree Maker:*		
Barbecued:		
Without chicken	3.1 oz.	150
*With chicken	6.8 oz.	320
Sweet & sour:		
Without chicken	4.1 oz.	130
*With chicken	7.8 oz.	300
(Swanson) & dumplings	7½ oz.	220
Frozen:		
(Armour):		
Classics Lite:		
Burgundy	10-oz. dinner	210
Marsala	10½-oz.	250
Sweet & sour	11-oz. dinner	240
Dining Lite, glazed	9-oz. meal	220
Dinner Classics:		
Glazed	10¾-oz. meal	300
Parmigiana	11¼-oz. meal	370
Dinner:		
Regular:		
& dumplings	10-oz. dinner	430
Fried	10-oz. dinner	400
Extra Helping:		
Fried, all white meat	16-oz. dinner	570
Nuggets, with sweet & sour sauce	10-oz. dinner	650
Family Entree:		
& dumplings	¼ of 28-oz. pkg.	280
& vegetable primavera	¼ of 28-oz. pkg.	140
(Healthy Balance):		
Mesquite	10½-oz. meal	310
Parmesan	10.8-oz. meal	300
Sweet & sour	10¼-oz. meal	270
Platter:		
Boneless, pattie	7½-oz. meal	380
Fried, all white meat, hot 'n spicy	9-oz. meal	430
(Budget Gourmet):		
Regular:		
Cacciatore, three-dish	11-oz. meal	300

Food and Description	Measure or Quantity	Calories
& egg noodles	10-oz. meal	450
With fettucini	10-oz. meal	400
Slim Selects:		
Au gratin	9.1-oz. meal	260
French recipe	10-oz. meal	260
Mandarin	10-oz. meal	290
(Celentano):		
Parmigiana	9-oz. meal	400
Primavera	11½-oz. pkg.	260
(Chun King) & walnuts, crunchy	13-oz. meal	310
(Healthy Choice):		
A l'orange	9½-oz. meal	260
Herb roasted	11-oz. meal	260
Mesquite	10½-oz. meal	310
Sweet & sour	11½-oz. meal	280
(Kid Cuisine):		
Fried	7¼-oz. meal	425
Nuggets	8.4-oz. meal	470
(La Choy) *Fresh & Lite*:		
Almond with rice and		
vegetables	9⅜-oz. meal	270
Oriental, spicy	9⅜-oz. meal	270
(Le Menu):		
Regular:		
Cordon bleu	11-oz. dinner	460
Sweet & sour	11¼-oz. dinner	400
Healthy dinner:		
Glazed breast	10-oz. dinner	230
Sweet & sour	10-oz. dinner	250
(Morton):		
Regular:		
Boneless	11-oz. dinner	329
Fried	11-oz. pkg.	431
Light, boneless	11-oz. dinner	250
(Stouffer's):		
Regular:		
Cashew in sauce, with rice	9½-oz. meal	380
Divan	8½-oz. meal	320
Dinner Supreme:		
Barbecue-style	10½ oz. meal	390
Florentine	11-oz. meal	430
Fried	10⅝-oz. meal	450
Parmigiana	11½-oz. meal	360
Lean Cuisine:		
Glazed; with vegetable rice	8½-oz. serving	270
& vegetables with vermicelli	12¾-oz. serving	260

Food and Description	Measure or Quantity	Calories
Right Course:		
Italiano, with fettucini & vegetables	9⅝-oz. meal	280
Sesame	10-oz. meal	320
Tenderloin, in barbecue sauce with rice pilaf	8¾-oz. meal	270
(Swanson):		
Regular:		
Fried:		
BBQ flavor	10-oz. dinner	540
White meat	10¼-oz. dinner	550
Nuggets	8¾-oz dinner	470
Homestyle Recipe, entrees:		
Cacciatore	10.9-oz. entree	260
Nibbles	4¼-oz. entree	340
Hungry Man, dinner:		
Boneless	17¾-oz. dinner	700
Fried, white meat	14¼-oz. dinner	870
(Tyson):		
Healthy Portion:		
BBQ	12½-oz. meal	470
Herb	13¾-oz. meal	340
Salsa	13¾-oz. meal	370
Sesame	13½-oz. meal	390
Loony Tunes:		
Drummetes, *Tasmanian Devil*	1 serving	310
Glazed, BBQ, *Yosemite Sam*	1 serving	230
Premium Dinner:		
Francais	9½-oz. meal	280
Honey roasted	9-oz. meal	220
Kiev	9¼-oz. meal	520
Picante	9-oz. meal	250
Ultra Slim Fast:		
Fettucini	12-oz. meal	390
Mesquite	12-oz. meal	360
Roasted, with mushrooms	12-oz. meal	280
Sweet & sour	12-oz. meal	330
& vegetables	12-oz. meal	290
(Weight Watchers):		
Regular:		
Fettucini	8¼-oz. meal	280
Polynesian	9-oz. meal	190
Sesame, with noodles	9-oz. meal	200
Smart Ones:		
Fiesta	8-oz. meal	210

Food and Description	Measure or Quantity	Calories
Lemon herb picatta	7½-oz. meal	160
Stir fry:		
Polynesian	9-oz. meal	190
Sesame	9-oz. meal	200
Ultimate 200:		
Barbecue glazed	7-oz. meal	200
Cordon bleu	7.7-oz. meal	170
Kiev	7-oz. meal	190
Southern baked	6.3-oz. meal	170
Mix (Lipton) *Microeasy:*		
Barbecue	¼ pkg.	108
Country	¼ pkg.	78
*Refrigerated, *Perdue Done It!*:		
Breast:		
Cutlets	3 oz.	210
Nuggets:		
Cheese	3 oz.	243
Fun shaped	3 oz.	222
Original	3 oz.	210
Tenders	3 oz.	189
Roasted:		
Regular	3 oz.	138
Cornish game hen	3 oz.	134
Wings:		
Barbecued	3 oz.	195
Garlic butter & herb	3 oz.	186
Hot & spicy	3 oz.	180
CHICKEN, FRIED, frozen:		
(Banquet):		
Assorted	32-oz. pkg.	1,650
Breast portion	11½-oz. pkg.	440
Hot 'n spicy, thigh & drumstick	12½-oz. meal	500
(Country Pride) southern fried, patties	3 oz.	232
(Swanson)		
Assorted	3¼-oz. serving	270
Breast portions	4½-oz. serving	360
Nibbles	3¼-oz. serving	300
***CHICKEN HELPER** (General Mills):		
Crispy, & biscuits	1 serving	710
Mushroom	1 serving	470
Tetrazzini	1 serving	320
CHICKEN & NOODLES, frozen:		
(Armour):		
Dining Lite	9-oz. meal	240
Dinner Classics	11-oz. meal	230

Food and Description	Measure or Quantity	Calories
(Stouffer's):		
Escalloped	5¾-oz. serving	252
Paprikash	10½-oz. serving	391
(Weight Watchers) homestyle	9-oz. meal	240
CHICKEN NUGGETS, frozen		
(See also CHICKEN DINNER OR		
ENTREE; HOT BITES; etc.):		
(Country Pride)	¼ of 12-oz. pkg.	250
(Empire Kosher)	¼ of 12-oz. pkg.	177
(Swanson)	3 oz.	230
CHICKEN, PACKAGED:		
(Carl Buddig) smoked	1 oz.	60
(Louis Rich) breast, oven roasted	1-oz. slice	35
(Weaver):		
Bologna	1 slice	44
Breast, oven roasted	1 slice	25
Roll	1 slice	26
CHICKEN PATTY, frozen:		
(Country Pride):		
Regular	¼ of 12-oz. pkg.	250
Southern fried	¼ of 12-oz. pkg.	240
(Empire Kosher)	¼ of 12-oz. pkg.	198
(Tyson)	2.6-oz. serving	220
CHICKEN PIE, frozen:		
(Banquet) regular	8-oz. pie	550
(Empire Kosher)	8-oz. pie	463
(Stouffer's)	10-oz. pie	530
(Swanson) regular	7-oz. pie	380
CHICKEN SALAD (Carnation)	¼ of 7½-oz. can	94
CHICKEN SOUP (See SOUP,		
Chicken)		
CHICKEN SPREAD:		
(Hormel) regular	1 oz.	60
(Underwood) chunky	½ of 4⅜-oz. can	150
CHICKEN STEW, canned:		
Regular:		
(Libby's) with dumplings	8 oz.	194
(Swanson)	7¾ oz.	160
Dietetic (Featherweight)	7½-oz. serving	140
CHICKEN STICKS, frozen (Country		
Pride)	3 oz.	233
CHICKEN STOCK BASE (French's)	1 tsp.	8
CHICK-FIL-A:		
Brownie, fudge, with nuts	2.8-oz. piece	369
Chicken, no bun	3.6-oz. serving	219

Food and Description	Measure or Quantity	Calories
Chicken nuggets, 8-pack	4 oz.	287
Chicken salad:		
Regular:		
Cup	3.4-oz. serving	309
Plate	11.8-oz. serving	475
Chargrilled, golden	16.4-oz. serving	126
Sandwich, chargrilled	5½-oz. serving	258
Chicken sandwich, with bun:		
Regular	5⅜-oz. serving	360
Deluxe chargrilled, with lettuce & tomato	7.15-oz. serving	266
Coleslaw	3.7-oz. cup	175
Icedream	4½-oz. serving	135
Pie, lemon	4.1-oz. piece	329
Potato, *Waffle Potato Fries*	3-oz. serving	270
Potato salad	3.8-oz. serving	198
Salad, tossed:		
Plain	4½-oz. serving	21
With dressing:		
Honey french	6-oz. serving	246
Italian, light	6-oz. serving	46
1000 Island	6-oz. serving	231
Soup, hearty breast of chicken, small	8½-oz. serving	152
CHICK'N QUICK, frozen (Tyson):		
Breast fillet	3 oz.	190
Breast pattie	3 oz.	240
Chick'N Cheddar	3 oz.	260
Cordon bleu	5 oz.	310
Kiev	5 oz.	430
CHICK PEA OR GARBANZO,		
canned, solids & liq.:		
(Allen's; Goya)	½ cup	110
(A&P)	½ cup	100
(Progresso)	½ cup	120
(Town House)	½ cup	110
CHILI OR CHILI CON CARNE:		
Canned, regular pack:		
Beans only:		
(Allens) hot, regular	½ cup	90
(A&P) hot	½ cup	140
(Hormel) in sauce	5 oz.	130
(Hunt's)	1 cup	200
(Town House)	½ cup	110
(Van Camp) Mexican style	1 cup	210
With beans:		
(Gebhardt) hot	½ of 15-oz. can	470

Food and Description	Measure or Quantity	Calories
(Hormel):		
Regular, mild or hot	½ of 15-oz. can	310
Micro-Cup	7½-oz. serving	250
Top Shelf	1 serving	320
(Hunt's) *Just Rite*, hot	4 oz.	195
(Libby's)	7½-oz. serving	270
(Old El Paso)	1 cup	217
(Swanson)	7⅜-oz. serving	310
Without beans:		
(Gebhardt)	½ of 15-oz. can	410
(Hormel) regular or hot	7½-oz. serving	370
(Hunt's) *Just Rite*	4-oz. serving	180
(Libby's)	7½ oz.	390
With chicken (Hain) spicy	7½-oz. serving	130
Vegetarian:		
With beans (Health Valley)	½ cup	130
Without beans (Gebhardt)	½ cup	219
Canned, dietetic pack:		
(Estee) with beans	7½-oz. serving	370
(Featherweight) with beans	7½ oz.	280
Frozen (Stouffer's):		
Regular, with beans	8¾-oz. meal	260
Right Choice, vegetarian	9¾-oz. meal	280
*Mix, *Manwich, Chili Fixins*	8 oz.	290
CHILI SAUCE:		
(Del Monte)	¼ cup (2 oz.)	70
(El Molino) green, mild	1 T.	5
(Heinz)	1 T.	17
(La Victoria)	1 T.	16
(Ortega) green, medium	1 oz.	7
(Featherweight) dietetic	1 T.	8
CHILI SEASONING MIX:		
*(Durkee)	1 cup	465
(French's) *Chili-O*, plain	1¾-oz. pkg.	150
(Lawry's)	1.6-oz. pkg.	143
(McCormick)	1.2-oz. pkg.	106
CHIMICHANGA, frozen:		
Marquez (Fred's Frozen Foods), beef, shredded	5-oz. serving	351
(Old El Paso):		
Regular, chicken	1 piece	360
Dinner, festive, beef	11-oz. dinner	540
Entree, bean & cheese	1 piece	350
CHOCOLATE, BAKING:		
(Baker's):		
Milk, chips	1 oz.	152

Food and Description	Measure or Quantity	Calories
Semi-sweet:		
Chocolate flavored:		
Chips	¼ cup	212
Square	1 oz.	150
Real	¼ cup	224
Sweetened, *German's*:		
Chips	¼ cup	230
Square	1 oz.	158
(Hershey's):		
Bitter or unsweetened	1 oz.	190
Sweetened:		
Milk:		
Chips:		
Regular	1 oz.	150
Vanilla	1 oz.	160
Chunks	1 oz.	160
Semi-sweet:		
Bar or chunks	1 oz.	140
Chips	1 oz.	147
(Nestlé):		
Bitter or unsweetened, *Choco-bake*	1-oz. packet	180
Sweet or semi-sweet, morsels	1 oz.	150
*CHOCOLATE DRINK:		
Canned (Yoo-Hoo)	8 fl. oz.	130
Mix (Lucerne)	8 fl. oz.	240
CHOCOLATE ICE CREAM (See ICE CREAM, Chocolate)		
CHOCOLATE SYRUP (See SYRUP, Chocolate)		
CHOP SUEY, frozen (Stouffer's) beef with rice	12-oz. pkg.	340
*CHOP SUEY SEASONING MIX (Durkee)	1¾ cups	557
CHOWDER (See SOUP, Chowder)		
CHOW MEIN:		
Canned:		
(Chun King) Divider-Pak:		
Beef	¼ pkg.	91
Chicken	½ of 24-oz. pkg.	110
Shrimp	¼ pkg.	91
(Hormel) pork, *Short Orders*	7½-oz. can	140
(La Choy):		
Regular:		
Beef	¾ cup	60
Chicken	¾ cup	70

Food and Description	Measure or Quantity	Calories
Shrimp	¾ cup	45
*Bi-pack:		
Beef	¾ cup	70
Beef pepper oriental, chicken or shrimp	¾ cup	80
Vegetable	¾ cup	50
Frozen:		
(Armour) *Dining Lite,* chicken & rice	9-oz. dinner	180
(Chun King) chicken	13-oz. entree	370
(Empire Kosher)	½ of 15-oz. pkg.	97
(Healthy Choice)	8½-oz. meal	220
(La Choy):		
Chicken	12-oz. dinner	260
Shrimp	12-oz. dinner	220
(Stouffer's) *Lean Cuisine,* with rice	11¼-oz. serving	250
CHOW MEIN SEASONING MIX (Kikkoman)	1⅛-oz. pkg.	98
CHURCH'S FRIED CHICKEN:		
Chicken, fried:		
Breast	4.3-oz. piece	278
Leg	2.9-oz. piece	147
Thigh	4.2-oz. piece	306
Wing-breast	4.8-oz. piece	303
Corn, with butter oil	1 ear	237
French-fried potatoes	1 regular order	138
CHUTNEY (Major Grey's)	1 T.	53
CINNAMON, GROUND (French's)	1 tsp.	6
CINNAMON TOAST CRUNCH, cereal (General Mills)	¾ cup	120
CITRUS BERRY BLEND, mix, dietctic (Sunkist)	8 fl. oz.	6
CITRUS COOLER DRINK, canned:		
(Five Alive)	6 fl. oz.	87
(Hi-C)	6 fl. oz.	95
CLAM:		
Raw, all kinds, meat only	1 cup (8 oz.)	186
Raw, soft, meat & liq.	1 lb. (weighed in shell)	142
Canned:		
(Doxsee):		
Chopped, minced or whole:		
Solids & liquid	½ cup	97
Drained solids	½ cup	58
(Gorton's) minced, meat only	1 can	140

Food and Description	Measure or Quantity	Calories
Frozen:		
(Gorton's) strips, crunchy, Microwave Specialty	3½ oz.	330
(Howard Johnson's)	5-oz. pkg.	395
(Mrs. Paul's) fried, light	2½-oz. serving	200
CLAM JUICE (Snow)	½ cup	15
CLAMATO COCKTAIL (Mott's)	6 fl. oz.	96
CLARET WINE:		
(Gold Seal) 12% alcohol	3 fl. oz.	82
(Taylor) 12.5% alcohol	3 fl. oz.	72
CLORETS, gum or mint	1 piece	6
CLUSTERS, cereal		
(General Mills)	½ cup	110
COBBLER, frozen (Pet-Ritz):		
Apple or strawberry	⅙ of 26-oz. pkg.	290
Blackberry	⅙ of 26-oz. pkg.	270
Cherry	⅙ of 26-oz. pkg.	280
Peach	⅙ of 26-oz. pkg.	260
COCKTAIL (See individual listings such as DAIQUIRI; PIÑA COLADA; etc.)		
COCOA:		
Dry, unsweetened:		
(Hershey's) regular	1 T.	22
(Sultana)	1 T.	30
Mix, regular:		
(Alba '66) instant, all flavors	1 envelope	60
(Carnation) all flavors	1-oz. pkg.	110
(Hershey's) instant	3 T.	81
(Ovaltine) hot 'n rich	1 oz.	120
(Pathmark) with mini marshmallows	1 oz.	110
Swiss Miss, regular or with mini marshmallows	6 fl. oz.	110
Mix, dietetic:		
(Carnation):		
70 Calorie	¾-oz. packet	70
*Sugar free	6 fl. oz.	50
(Lucerne)	1 envelope	50
Swiss Miss, instant, lite	1 envelope	70
(Weight Watchers)	1 envelope	60
COCOA KRISPIES, cereal		
(Kellogg's)	¾ cup (1 oz.)	110
COCOA PUFFS, cereal		
(General Mills)	1 cup (1 oz.)	110
COCONUT:		
Fresh, meat only	2" × 2" × ½" piece	156

Food and Description	Measure or Quantity	Calories
Grated or shredded, loosely packed	½ cup	225
Dried:		
(Baker's):		
Angel Flake	⅓ cup	118
Cookie	⅓ cup	186
Premium shred	⅓ cup	138
(Town House) flaked or shredded	1 oz.	150
COCONUT, CREAM OF, canned:		
(Coco Lopez)	1 T.	60
(Holland House)	1 oz.	81
COCO WHEATS, cereal (Little Crow)	1 T.	43
COD:		
Broiled	3 oz.	145
Frozen:		
(Captain's Choice) fillet	3 oz.	89
(Frionor) *Norway Gourmet*	4-oz. fillet	70
(Van de Kamp's) *Natural*	4-oz.	90
COD DINNER OR ENTREE, frozen:		
(Armour) *Dinner Classics,* almondine	12-oz. dinner	360
(Frionor) *Norway Gourmet,* with dill sauce	4½-oz. fillet	80
(Mrs. Paul's) light	1 piece	240
(Van de Kamp's) breaded, light	1 piece	250
COD LIVER OIL (Hain)	1 T.	120
COFFEE:		
Regular:		
Max-Pax; Maxwell House Electra Perk; Yuban, Yuban Electra Matic	6 fl. oz.	2
Mellow Roast	6 fl.oz.	8
Decaffeinated:		
Brim, regular or electric perk	6 fl. oz.	2
Sanka, regular or electric perk	6 fl. oz.	2
*Instant:		
Regular:		
Maxwell House; Taster's Choice	6 fl. oz.	4
Mellow Roast	6 fl. oz.	8
Sunrise	6 fl. oz.	6
Decaffeinated:		
Brim, freeze-dried; *Decafé; Nescafé*	6 fl. oz.	4

Food and Description	Measure or Quantity	Calories
*Mix (General Foods) *International Coffee:*		
Café Amaretto, Café Français	6 fl. oz.	59
Café Vienna, Orange Cappuccino	6 fl. oz.	65
Suisse Mocha	6 fl. oz.	58
COFFEE CAKE (See CAKE, Coffee)		
COFFEE LIQUEUR (DeKuyper)	1½ fl. oz.	140
COFFEE SOUTHERN	1 fl. oz.	79
COGNAC (See DISTILLED LIQUOR)		
COLA SOFT DRINK (See SOFT DRINK, Cola)		
COLD DUCK WINE (Lejon) pink	3 fl. oz.	81
COLESLAW, solids & liq., made with mayonnaise-type salad dressing	1 cup	119
***COLESLAW MIX** (Libby's)*		
Super Slaw	½ cup	240
COLLARDS:		
Leaves, cooked	⅓ pkg.	31
Canned (Allen's) chopped, solids & liq.	½ cup	25
Frozen:		
(Bel-Air)	3.3 oz.	25
(Birds Eye) chopped	⅓ pkg.	30
(Southland) chopped	⅕ of 16-oz. pkg.	25
COMPLETE CEREAL (Elam's)	1 oz.	109
CONCORD WINE:		
(Gold Seal)	3 fl. oz.	125
(Pleasant Valley) red	3 fl. oz.	90
COOKIE, REGULAR:		
Angelica Goodies (Stella D'oro)	1 piece	110
Angel Wings (Stella D'oro)	1 piece	70
Anginetti (Stella D'oro)	1 piece	30
Animal:		
(Dixie Belle)	1 piece	8
(FFV)	1 piece	14
(Nabisco) *Barnum's Animals*	1 piece	12
(Sunshine)	1 piece	8
(Tom's)	½ oz.	62
Anisette sponge (Stella D'oro)	1 piece	50
Anisette toast (Stella D'oro):		
Regular	1 piece	50

Food and Description	Measure or Quantity	Calories
Jumbo	1 piece	110
Apple N' Raisin (Archway)	1 cookie	120
Apricot Raspberry (Pepperidge Farm)	1 piece	50
Assortment:		
(Nabisco) *Mayfair:*		
Crown creme sandwich	1 piece	53
Fancy shortbread biscuit	1 piece	22
Filigree creme sandwich	1 piece	60
Mayfair creme sandwich	1 piece	65
Tea rose creme	1 piece	53
(Stella D'oro) hostess or *Lady Stella*	1 piece	40
Blueberry Newtons (Nabisco)	1 piece	73
Bordeaux (Pepperidge Farm)	1 piece	35
Breakfast Treats (Stella D'oro)	1 piece	100
Brown edge wafer (Nabisco)	1 piece	28
Brownie:		
(Hostess)	1.25-oz. piece	157
(Little Debbie) fudge	2-oz. piece	240
(Nabisco) *Almost Home*	1¼-oz. piece	160
(Pepperidge Farm) chocolate nut	.4-oz. piece	55
(Tastybake) walnut	3-oz. piece	335
(Weight Watchers) chocolate, frozen	⅓ of pkg.	100
Brussels (Pepperidge Farm:		
Regular	1 piece	55
Mint	1 piece	65
Butter (Sunshine)	1 piece	30
Cappuccino (Pepperidge Farm)	1 piece	50
Caramel Patties (FFV)	1 piece	75
Castelets (Stella D'oro)	1 piece	70
Checkerboard wafer (Mother's)	1 piece	17
Chessman (Pepperidge Farm)	1 piece	45
Chocolate & chocolate-covered:		
(Keebler) stripes	1 piece	50
(Nabisco):		
Pinwheel, cake	1 piece	130
Snap	1 piece	19
(Sunshine) nuggets	1 piece	23
Chocolate chip:		
(Archway) regular	1 piece	110
(Famous Amos):		
With nuts, macadamia	1 oz.	152
Without nuts, extra chips	1 oz.	147
(Frookie) regular or mandarin orange	1 piece	45

Food and Description	Measure or Quantity	Calories
(Keebler) Rich 'n Chips	1 piece	80
(Mother's):		
Regular	1 piece	70
Angel	1 piece	60
Oatmeal walnut	1 piece	70
(Nabisco):		
Almost Home	1 piece	65
Chips Ahoy!:		
Regular	1 piece	47
Chewy	1 piece	60
Sprinkled	1 piece	60
Striped	1 piece	90
Snaps	1 piece	22
(Pepperidge Farm):		
Regular	1 piece	50
Chesapeake	1 piece	120
Nantucket	1 piece	120
Pecan	1 piece	70
(Sunshine):		
Chip-A-Roos	1 piece	60
Chippy Chews	1 piece	50
(Tom's)	1.7-oz. serving	230
Coconut fudge (FFV)	1 piece	80
Como Delights (Stella D'oro)	1 piece	150
Dinosaurs (FFV)	1 oz.	130
Dutch apple bar (Stella D'oro)	1 piece	110
Dutch cocoa (Archway)	1 piece	110
Egg biscuit (Stella D'oro):		
Regular	1 piece	80
Roman	1 piece	140
Egg jumbo (Stella D'oro)	1 piece	50
Fig bar:		
(FFV)	1 piece	70
(Mother's):		
Regular	1 bar	55
(Nabisco) *Fig Newtons*	1 piece	50
(Sunshine) Chewies	1 piece	50
(Tom's)	1.8-oz. serving	170
Fruit Stick (Nabisco) *Almost Home*	1 piece	70
Fudge (Stella D'oro) swiss	1 piece	70
Geneva (Pepperidge Farm)	1 piece	65
Gingerman (Pepperidge Farm)	1 piece	35
Ginger snap:		
(Archway)	1 piece	25
(FFV)	1 oz.	130
(Nabisco)	1 piece	30
(Sunshine)	1 piece	20

Food and Description	Measure or Quantity	Calories
Ginger Spice (Frookie)	1 piece	45
Golden bars (Stella D'oro)	1 piece	110
Golden fruit raisin (Sunshine)	1 piece	70
Hazelnut (Pepperidge Farm)	1 piece	55
Jelly tarts (FFV)	1 piece	60
Ladyfinger	3¼" × 1⅜" × 1⅛"	40
Lido (Pepperidge Farm)	1 piece	90
Linzer (Pepperidge Farm)	1 piece	120
Macaroon, coconut (Nabisco)	1 piece	95
Mallow Puffs (Sunshine)	1 piece	70
Margherite (Stella D'oro)	1 piece	70
Marshmallow:		
(Nabisco):		
Mallomars	1 piece	65
Puffs, cocoa covered	1 piece	120
Sandwich	1 piece	30
Twirls cakes	1 piece	130
(Planters) banana pie	1 oz.	127
Milano (Pepperidge Farm):		
Regular	1 piece	60
Mint or orange	1 piece	75
Molasses:		
(Archway)	1 piece	100
(Nabisco) *Pantry*	1 piece	65
Molasses crisp (Pepperidge Farm)	1 piece	35
Nilla wafer (Nabisco)	1 piece	19
Oatmeal:		
(Archway):		
Regular	1 piece	110
Date filled	1 piece	100
(Famous Amos) with cinnamon &		
raisins	1 oz.	133
(FFV) bar	1 piece	70
(Keebler) old fashioned	1 piece	80
(Mother's):		
Chocolate chip, with or without		
walnuts	1 piece	70
Iced	1 piece	70
Raisin	1 piece	32
(Nabisco) *Bakers Bonus*	1 piece	65
(Pepperidge Farm):		
Irish	1 piece	45
Raisin, regular	1 piece	55
(Sunshine) country	1 piece	60
Orbits (Sunshine)	1 piece	15
Peach apricot bar (FFV)	1 piece	70

Food and Description	Measure or Quantity	Calories
Peanut & peanut butter (Nabisco):		
Almost Home	1 piece	70
Nutter Butter, sandwich	1 piece	70
Pecan Sandies (Keebler)	1 piece	80
Pfenernusse (Stella D'oro)	1 piece	40
Raisin:		
(Nabisco) *Almost Home:*		
Fudge chocolate chip	1 piece	65
Iced applesauce	1 piece	70
(Pepperidge Farm) bran	1 piece	53
Raisin bran (Pepperidge Farm)		
Kitchen Hearth	1 piece	55
Raspberry filled (Archway)	1 cookie	105
Rocky road (Archway)	1 cookie	130
Royal Dainty (FFV)	1 piece	60
Sandwich:		
(FFV) mint	1 piece	80
(Keebler):		
Fudge creme	1 piece	60
Pitter Patter	1 piece	90
(Mother's):		
Double fudge	1 piece	50
Duplex	1 piece	52
English tea	1 piece	100
Peanut butter, *Gaucho*	1 piece	90
(Nabisco):		
Almost Home	1 piece	140
Baronet	1 piece	47
Gaity	1 piece	50
Giggles	1 piece	70
I Screams	1 piece	75
Oreo, regular	1 piece	47
(Sunshine):		
Regular, *Hydrox*	1 piece	50
Chips 'n Middles	1 piece	70
Tru Blu	1 piece	80
Sesame (Stella D'oro)		
Regina	1 piece	50
Shortbread or shortcake:		
(FFV) country	1 piece	70
(Nabisco):		
Lorna Doone	1 piece	35
Pecan	1 piece	75
(Pepperidge Farm) pecan	1 piece	70
Social Tea, biscuit (Nabisco)	1 piece	22
Sprinkles (Sunshine)	1 piece	70

Food and Description	Measure or Quantity	Calories
Sugar cookie (Nabisco) rings, *Bakers Bonus*	1 piece	65
Sugar wafer:		
(Dutch Twin) any flavor	1 piece	36
(Nabisco) *Biscos*	1 piece	19
(Sunshine)	1 piece	45
Tahiti (Pepperidge Farm)	1 piece	90
Toy (Sunshine)	1 piece	12
Vanilla wafer (FFV)	1 piece	130
Waffle creme (Dutch Twin)	1 piece	45
COOKIE, DIETETIC:		
Animal (Health Valley) oat bran	1 oz.	90
Amaranth (Health Valley)	1 piece	60
Apple (Health Valley) with fruit center, fat free	1 piece	23
Apple pastry (Stella D'oro)	1 piece	90
Apple Spice (Health Valley) fat free	1 piece	25
Apricot Almond Fancy Fruit Chunks (Health Valley)	1 piece	30
Apricot with fruit center (Health Valley) fat free	1 piece	23
Chocolate Chip:		
(Estee)	1 piece	36
(Featherweight):		
Regular	1 piece	40
Double	1 piece	45
Coconut:		
(Estee)	1 piece	30
(Stella D'oro)	1 piece	50
Date Delight (Health Valley) fat free	1 piece	25
Date with fruit center (Health Valley)	1 piece	23
Egg biscuit (Stella D'oro)	1 piece	40
Fruit & Fitness (Health Valley)	1 oz.	100
Fruit & Honey (Entenmann's)	1 piece	40
Fruit Bar (Health Valley):		
Regular, Apple Bakes	1 bar	82
Fat free, any flavor	1 bar	140
Jumbo	1 bar	140
Fudge (Estee)	1 piece	30
Graham, healthy (Health Valley) any flavor	1 oz.	110
Hawaiian Fruit (Health Valley) fat free	1 piece	25
Kichel (Stella D'oro)	1 piece	8
Lemon (Featherweight)	1 piece	40

Food and Description	Measure or Quantity	Calories
Oatmeal raisin:		
(Entenmann's)	1 piece	40
(Estee)	1 piece	30
(Featherweight)	1 piece	45
Prune pastry (Stella D'oro)	1 piece	90
Sandwich (Estee) original	1 piece	45
Sesame (Stella D'oro) Regina	1 piece	40
Wafer, creme:		
(Estee):		
Assorted	1 piece	30
Chocolate or Vanilla	1 piece	20
(Featherweight):		
Chocolate or strawberry	1 piece	20
Peanut butter	1 piece	25
Wafer, snack (Estee)	1 piece	80
Wafer, vanilla (Featherweight)	1 piece	30
COOKIE CRISP, cereal, any flavor		
(Ralston Purina)	1 cup	110
*COOKIE DOUGH:		
Refrigerated (Pillsbury):		
Brownie, microwave, with chocolate chips	1 piece	180
Oatmeal raisin or peanut butter	1 cookie	70
Frozen (Rich's):		
Chocolate chip	1 cookie	138
Oatmeal	1 cookie	125
COOKIE MIX:		
Regular:		
Brownie:		
*(Betty Crocker):		
Chocolate chip	½₄ of pan	130
Frosted	½₄ of pan	160
Fudge, family size	½₄ of pan	130
Walnut	½₄ of pan	140
(Duncan Hines):		
Chewy	½₄ pkg.	98
Fudge, original	½₄ pkg.	122
Peanut butter	½₄ pkg.	120
Truffle	⅟₁₆ pkg.	200
*(Gold Medal) fudge	⅟₁₆ pkg.	100
*(Pillsbury) fudge:		
Regular	2" sq. (⅟₁₆ pkg.)	150
Microwave	⅛ of pkg.	190
Ultimate, rocky road	2" sq. (⅟₁₆ of pkg.)	170
Chocolate chip:		
*(Betty Crocker) *Big Batch*	1 cookie	60
*(Duncan Hines)	⅟₃₆ pkg.	73

Food and Description	Measure or Quantity	Calories
*(Quaker)	1 cookie	75
*Fudge chip (Quaker)	1 cookie	75
*Macaroon, coconut (Betty Crocker)	⅟₂₄ pkg.	80
Oatmeal (Duncan Hines) raisin	⅟₃₆ pkg.	68
Peanut butter (Duncan Hines)	⅟₃₆ pkg.	68
Sugar (Duncan Hines)	1 cookie	59
Dietetic (Estee) brownie	2" × 2" sq. cookie	45
COOKING SPRAY:		
Mazola No Stick	2½-second spray	6
Pam	2½-second spray	2
(Weight Watchers)	2½-second spray	5
Wesson Lite	2-second spray	<1
CORN:		
Fresh, on the cob, boiled	5" × 1⅜" ear	70
Canned, regular pack, solids & liq.:		
(Allen's) whole kernel	½ cup	80
(A&P)	½ cup	80
(Comstock) whole kernel	½ cup	90
(Green Giant):		
Cream style	4¼ oz.	100
Whole kernel, golden	4¼ oz.	80
Whole kernel, *Mexicorn*	3½ oz.	80
(Larsen) *Freshlike,* whole kernel, vacuum pack	½ cup	100
(Libby's) cream style	½ cup	100
(Pathmark) No Frills	½ cup	80
(Stokely-Van Camp):		
Cream style	½ cup	105
Whole kernel, solids & liq.	½ cup	74
(Town House) cream style	½ cup	80
Canned, dietetic pack, solids & liq.:		
(A&P)	½ cup	80
(Diet Delight)	½ cup	60
(Green Giant)	½ cup	80
(Larsen) *Fresh-Lite*	½ cup	80
(Pathmark)	½ cup	70
(S&W) *Nutradiet,* whole kernel, green label	½ cup	80
Frozen:		
(Bel-Air):		
On the cob, regular	1 ear	120
Whole kernel	3.3 oz.	80
(Birds Eye):		
On the cob:		
Regular	4.4-oz. ear	120
Little Ears	4.6-oz. ear	126

Food and Description	Measure or Quantity	Calories
With butter sauce	⅓ pkg.	85
(Budget Gourmet) in butter sauce	5½ oz.	190
(Frosty Acres):		
On the cob	1 whole ear	120
Kernels	3.3 oz.	80
(Green Giant):		
On the cob, regular:		
Nibbler	1 ear	60
Niblet ear	1 ear	120
Whole kernel, butter sauce, golden	4 oz.	100
Whole kernel, *Niblets,* golden, polybag	⅓ pkg.	80
(Health Valley) kernels	5.8 oz.	134
(Larsen):		
On the cob	3" piece (2.2 oz.)	60
Kernels	3.3 oz.	80
(Ore-Ida) cob corn	5.3-oz. ear	160
(Seabrook Farms):		
On the cob	5" ear	140
Whole kernel	⅓ pkg.	97
CORNBREAD:		
Home recipe:		
Corn pone	4 oz.	231
Spoon bread	4 oz.	221
*Mix:		
(Aunt Jemima)	⅙ pkg.	220
Gold Medal (General Mills)	⅙ pkg.	150
(Pillsbury) *Ballard*	⅛ of recipe	140
*CORN DOGS, frozen		
(Hormel)	1 piece	220
CORNED BEEF:		
Cooked, boneless, medium fat	4-oz. serving	422
Canned, regular pack:		
Dinty Moore (Hormel)	2-oz. serving	130
(Libby's)	⅓ of 7-oz. can	160
Canned, dietetic (Featherweight) loaf	2½-oz. serving	90
Packaged (Carl Buddig) sliced	1-oz. slice	40
CORNED BEEF HASH, canned:		
(Libby's)	⅓ of 24-oz. can	420
Mary Kitchen (Hormel)	7½-oz. serving	360
CORNED BEEF HASH DINNER,		
frozen (Banquet)	10-oz. dinner	372
CORNED BEEF SPREAD		
(Underwood)	½ of 4½-oz. can	120

Food and Description	Measure or Quantity	Calories
CORN FLAKE CRUMBS		
(Kellogg's)	¼ cup	100
CORN FLAKES, cereal:		
(General Mills) *Country*	1 cup (1 oz.)	110
(Kellogg's) regular	1 cup (1 oz.)	110
(Malt-O-Meal) sugar-coated	⅜ cup	109
(Ralston Purina) regular	1 cup	110
(Safeway) regular	1 cup	110
CORN MEAL:		
Bolted (Aunt Jemima/Quaker)	3 T.	102
Degermed	¼ cup	125
Mix, bolted (Aunt Jemima) white	1 cup	392
CORN POPS, cereal		
(Kellogg's)	1 cup	110
CORN PUREE (Larsen)	½ cup	100
CORNSTARCH (Argo; Kingsford's; Duryea)	1 tsp.	10
CORN SYRUP (See SYRUP, Corn)		
COUGH DROP:		
(Beech-Nut)	1 drop	10
(Pine Bros.)	1 drop	10
COUNT CHOCULA, cereal		
(General Mills)	1 cup (1 oz.)	110
*COUSCOUS MIX (Fantastic Foods)		
regular	½ cup	105
CRAB:		
Fresh, steamed:		
Whole	½ lb.	101
Meat only	4 oz.	105
Canned, drained	4 oz.	115
Frozen (Wakefield's), snow	4 oz.	96
CRAB, DEVILED, frozen		
(Mrs. Paul's) breaded & fried, regular	1 cake	180
CRAB, IMITATION (Louis Kemp)		
Crab Delights, chunks, flakes or legs	2 oz.	60
CRAB APPLE, flesh only	¼ lb.	71
CRAB APPLE JELLY (Smucker's)	1 T.	54
CRAB IMPERIAL, home recipe	1 cup	323
CRACKERS, PUFFS & CHIPS:		
Animal (FFV)	1 oz.	130
Arrowroot biscuit (Nabisco)	1 piece	22
Bacon-flavored thins (Nabisco)	1 piece	10
Bacon Nips	1 oz.	147
Bran wafer (Featherweight)	1 piece	13
Bravos (Wise)	1 oz.	150

Food and Description	Measure or Quantity	Calories
Bugles (Tom's)	1 oz.	150
Butter (Pepperidge Farm) thin	1 piece	17
Cafe (Sunshine)	1 piece	20
Cheese flavored:		
American Heritage (Sunshine):		
Cheddar	1 piece	16
Parmesan	1 piece	18
Better Blue Thins (Nabisco)	1 piece	7
Cheddar sticks (Flavor Tree)	1 oz.	160
Cheese bites (Tom's)	1½ oz.	200
Cheese Doodles (Wise):		
Crunchy	1 oz.	160
Puffed	1 oz.	150
Cheese Wheels (Health Valley)	1 oz.	140
Chee-Tos:		
Crunchy, regular	1 oz.	150
Puffed balls or puffs	1 oz.	160
Cheez Balls (Planters)	1 oz.	160
Cheez Curls (Planters)	1 oz.	160
Cheeze-It (Sunshine)	1 piece	6
Corn Cheese (Tom's) crunchy	1⅝ oz.	280
(Dixie Belle)	1 piece	6
(Eagle)	1 oz.	130
Nacho cheese cracker (Keebler)	1 piece	11
Nips (Nabisco)	1 piece	5
Tid-Bit (Nabisco)	1 piece	4
Chicken in a Biskit (Nabisco)	1 piece	11
Chipsters (Nabisco)	1 piece	2
Club cracker (Keebler)	1 piece	15
Corn chips:		
(Bachman) regular or BBQ	1 oz.	150
Dipsy Doodle (Wise)	1 oz.	160
(Featherweight) low sodium	1 oz.	170
(Flavor Tree)	1 oz.	150
Fritos:		
Regular	1 oz.	150
Chili cheese flavor	1 oz.	160
Happy Heart (TKI Foods)	⅜ oz.	40
Heart Lovers (TKI Foods)	⅜ oz.	40
Korkers (Nabisco)	1 piece	8
(Laura Scudder's)	1 oz.	160
(Tom's) regular	1 oz.	155
Corn Snackers (Weight Watchers)	.5 oz.	60
Corn Stick (Flavor Tree)	1 oz.	160
Creme Wafer Stick (Nabisco)	1 piece	47
Crown Pilot (Nabisco)	1 piece	70
Diggers (Nabisco)	1 piece	4

Food and Description	Measure or Quantity	Calories
English Water Biscuit (Pepperidge Farm)	1 piece	17
Escort (Nabisco)	1 piece	23
Flutters (Pepperidge Farm):		
Garden herb	¾ oz.	100
Toasted wheat	¾ oz.	110
French onion cracker (Nabisco)	1 piece	12
Goldfish (Pepperidge Farm):		
Thins, cheese	1 piece	12
Tiny:		
Cheddar cheese	1 oz.	120
Pizza flavored	1 oz.	130
Pretzel	1 oz.	110
Graham:		
Cinnamon Crisp (Keebler)	1 piece	17
(Dixie Belle) sugar-honey coated	1 piece	15
Flavor Kist (Schulze and Burch)		
sugar-honey coated	1 piece	57
(Health Valley) fancy honey	1 oz.	130
Honey Maid (Nabisco)	1 piece	30
(Mother's):		
Dinosaur Grrrahams,		
cinnamon	1 piece	80
Royal	1 piece	69
(Rokeach)	8 pieces	120
(Sunshine) cinnamon	1 piece	17
Graham, chocolate or cocoa-covered:		
(Keebler)	1 piece	40
(Nabisco)	1 piece	57
Great Snackers (Weight Watchers)	.5-oz. pkg.	60
Hi Ho (Sunshine)	1 piece	20
Meal Mates (Nabisco)	1 piece	23
Melba Toast (See MELBA TOAST)		
Milk Lunch Biscuit (Keebler)	1 piece	27
Mucho Macho Nacho, Flavor Kist (Schulze and Burch)	1 oz.	121
Nachips (Old El Paso)	1 piece	17
Nacho Rings (Tom's)	1 oz.	160
Oat thins (Nabisco)	1 piece	9
Ocean Crisp (FFV)	1 piece	60
Onion rings (Wise)	1 oz.	130
Oyster:		
(Dixie Belle)	1 piece	4
(Keebler) *Zesta*	1 piece	2
(Nabisco) *Dandy* or *Oysterettes*	1 piece	3

Food and Description	Measure or Quantity	Calories
(Sunshine)	1 piece	4
Party mix (Flavor Tree)	1 oz.	160
Peanut butter & cheese (Eagle)	1.8-oz. serving	280
Pizza Crunchies (Planters)	1 oz.	160
Ritz (Nabisco)	1 piece	17
Ritz Bits (Nabisco):		
Regular, cheese or low salt	1 piece	3
Cheese sandwich or peanut butter		
sandwich	1 piece	13
Royal Lunch (Nabisco)	1 piece	60
Rye toast (Keebler)	1 piece	16
RyKrisp:		
Natural	1 triple cracker	20
Seasoned	1 triple cracker	22
Saltine:		
(Dixie Belle) regular or unsalted	1 piece	12
Krispy (Sunshine)	1 piece	12
Premium (Nabisco):		
Regular, low salt, unsalted tops		
or *Premium Plus* whole		
wheat	1 piece	12
Bits	1 piece	4
Fat free	1 piece	10
(Rokeach)	1 piece	12
Zesta (Keebler)	1 piece	12
Schooners (FFV) whole wheat	½ oz.	70
Sea Toast (Keebler)	1 piece	60
Sesame:		
American Heritage (Sunshine)	1 piece	17
Chip (Flavor Tree)	1 oz.	150
Crunch (Flavor Tree)	1 oz.	150
(Estee)	½ oz.	70
Stick (Flavor Tree):		
Regular	1 oz.	150
With bran or low sodium	1 oz.	160
Toast (Keebler)	1 piece	16
Sesame wheat (Natures Cupboard)	1 piece	11
Skittle Chips (Nabisco)	1 piece	14
Snackers (Ralston Purina)	1 piece	17
Snackin Crisp (Durkee) *D&C*	1 oz.	155
Snacks Sticks (Pepperidge Farm):		
Pretzel	1 piece	15
Pumpernickel	1 piece	17
Three cheese	1 piece	16
Sociables (Nabisco)	1 piece	12

Food and Description	Measure or Quantity	Calories
Sour cream-onion stick (Flavor Tree)	1 oz.	150
Spirals (Wise)	1 oz.	160
Stone ground (Natures Cupboard)	1 piece	11
Table Water Cracker (Carr's) small	1 piece	15
Taco chip (Laura Scudder's)	1 oz.	150
Tortilla chips:		
(Bachman) nacho, taco flavor or toasted	1 oz.	140
Doritos:		
Regular	1 oz.	140
Cool Ranch, light	1 oz.	120
Salsa Rio	1 oz.	140
(Eagle) *Del Masa*	1 oz.	150
(Laura Scudder's)	1 oz.	140
(Old El Paso)	1 oz.	150
(Planters)	1 oz.	150
(Tom's)	1½ oz.	210
Tostitos:		
Jalapeño & cheese	1 oz.	150
Traditional	1 oz.	140
Town House Cracker (Keebler)	1 piece	16
Triscuit (Nabisco) regular	1 piece	20
Tuc (Keebler)	1 piece	23
Twigs (Nabisco)	1 piece	14
Uneeda Biscuit (Nabisco) unsalted top	1 piece	30
Unsalted (Featherweight)	2 sections (½ cracker)	30
Waverly (Nabisco)	1 piece	17
Wheat:		
(Health Valley):		
Fat free, any flavor	½ oz.	40
No salt, stoned, herb, or sesame	½ oz.	55
(Keebler) *Wheatable,* any flavor	1 piece	6
(Pepperidge Farm):		
Cracked or hearty	1 piece	25
Toasted	1 piece	20
Wheatmeal Biscuit (Carr's) small	1 piece	42
Wheat Nuts (Flavor Tree)	1 oz.	200
Wheat Snack (Dixie Belle)	1 piece	9
Wheat Snax (Estee)	1 oz.	100
Wheat Snaz (Estee)	1 oz.	110
Wheatstone (Busy Baker)	1 piece	17
Wheatsworth (Nabisco)	1 piece	17

Food and Description	Measure or Quantity	Calories
Wheat Thins (Nabisco) nutty	1 piece	11
Wheat Toast (Keebler)	1 piece	15
CRACKER CRUMBS, graham:		
(Nabisco)	2 T.	80
(Sunshine)	½ cup	275
CRACKER MEAL (Nabisco)	2 T.	50
CRANAPPLE JUICE (Ocean Spray) canned:		
Regular	6 fl. oz.	127
Dietetic	6 fl. oz.	41
CRANBERRY, fresh (Ocean Spray)	½ cup	25
CRANBERRY APPLE DRINK, canned (Town House)	6 fl. oz.	130
CRANBERRY JUICE COCKTAIL:		
Canned (Ocean Spray):		
Regular	6 fl. oz.	103
Dietetic	6 fl. oz.	41
*Frozen (Sunkist)	6 fl. oz.	110
CRANBERRY-APPLE JUICE COCKTAIL, frozen (Welch's)	6 fl. oz.	120
CRANBERRY SAUCE:		
Home recipe, sweetened, unstrained	4 oz.	202
Canned (Ocean Spray):		
Jellied	2 oz.	87
Whole berry	2 oz.	93
CRAN-FRUIT (Ocean Spray)	2 oz.	100
CRANGRAPE (Ocean Spray)	6 fl. oz.	130
CRANRASPBERRY (Ocean Spray)	6 fl. oz.	110
CRANTASTIC JUICE DRINK, canned (Ocean Spray) regular	6 fl. oz.	110
CREAM:		
Half & half (Land O' Lakes)	1 T.	20
Heavy whipping:		
(Johanna Farms) 36% butterfat	1 T.	52
(Land O' Lakes) gourmet	1 T.	50
Light, table or coffee:		
(Johanna Farms) 18% butterfat	1 T.	30
(Sealtest) 16% butterfat	1 T.	26
Light, whipping, 30% fat (Sealtest)	1 T.	45
Sour:		
(Friendship):		
Regular	1 T.	27
Regular	½ cup	220
Light	1 oz.	35
(Johanna Farms)	1 T.	31

Food and Description	Measure or Quantity	Calories
(Land O' Lakes):		
Regular	1 T.	30
Light, plain or with chives	1 T.	20
(Lucerne) light	1 T.	22
(Weight Watchers) light	1 T.	17
Sour, imitation (Pet)	1 T.	25
Substitute (See CREAM SUBSTITUTE)		
CREAM PUFFS:		
Home recipe, custard filling	3½" × 2" piece	303
Frozen (Rich's) chocolate	1⅓-oz. piece	146
CREAM SUBSTITUTE:		
Coffee Mate (Carnation)	1 tsp.	11
Coffee Rich (Rich's)	½ oz.	22
Coffee Tone (Lucerne) non-dairy	½ fl. oz.	16
Cremora (Borden)	1 tsp.	12
Dairy Light (Alba)	2.8-oz. envelope	10
Mocha Mix (Presto Food Products)	1 T.	20
N-Rich	1 tsp.	10
(Pathmark) No Frills	1 tsp.	10
(Pet)	1 tsp.	10
CREAM OF RICE, cereal	1 oz.	100
CREAM OF WHEAT, cereal:		
Regular	1 oz.	100
*Instant	1 oz.	100
Mix'n Eat:		
Regular	1 packet	100
Apple & cinnamon	1 packet	130
Maple & brown sugar	1 packet	130
Quick	1 T.	40
CREME DE BANANA LIQUEUR (Mr. Boston)	1 fl. oz.	93
CREME DE CACAO:		
(Hiram Walker)	1 fl. oz.	104
(Mr. Boston):		
Brown	1 fl. oz.	102
White	1 fl. oz.	93
CREME DE CASSIS (Mr. Boston)	1 fl. oz.	85
CREME DE MENTHE:		
(Bols)	1 fl. oz.	122
(Mr. Boston):		
Green	1 fl. oz.	109
White	1 fl. oz.	97
CREME DE NOYAUX (Mr. Boston)	1 fl. oz.	99

Food and Description	Measure or Quantity	Calories
CREPE, frozen:		
(Mrs. Paul's):		
Crab	5½-oz. pkg.	248
Shrimp	5½-oz. pkg.	252
(Stouffer's):		
Chicken with mushroom sauce	8¼-oz. pkg.	390
Spinach with cheddar cheese sauce	9½-oz. pkg.	415
CRISP RICE CEREAL:		
(Malt-O-Meal) *Crisp 'N Crackling Rice*	1 cup	108
(Ralston Purina)	1 cup	110
(Safeway)	1 cup	110
CRISPY WHEATS'N RAISINS, cereal (General Mills)	¾ cup	110
CROUTON:		
(Arnold):		
Bavarian or English style	½ oz.	65
French, Italian or Mexican style	½ oz.	66
(Kellogg's) *Croutettes*	⅔ cup	70
(Mrs. Culberson's) cheese & garlic or seasoned	½ oz.	60
(Pepperidge Farm) cheese & garlic	½ oz.	70
CUCUMBER:		
Eaten with skin	8-oz. cucumber	32
Pared, whole	7½" × 2"	29
Pared, sliced	3 slices (.9 oz.)	4
CUMIN SEED (French's)	1 tsp.	7
***CUPCAKE MIX** (Flako)	1 cupcake	150
CURAÇAO LIQUEUR:		
(Bols)	1 fl. oz.	105
(Hiram Walker)	1 fl. oz.	96
CURRANT, DRIED (Del Monte) Zante	½ cup	204
CURRANT JELLY, sweetened		
(Home Brands)	1 T.	50
CUSTARD:		
Canned (Thank You Brand) egg	½ cup	135
Chilled, *Swiss Miss,* chocolate or egg flavor	4-oz. container	150
*Mix, dietetic (Featherweight)	½ cup	80
C. W. POST, cereal, hearty granola	¼ cup	128

Food and Description	Measure or Quantity	Calories

D

Food and Description	Measure or Quantity	Calories
DAIQUIRI COCKTAIL		
(Mr.Boston):		
Regular	3 fl. oz.	99
Strawberry	3 fl. oz.	111
***DAIQUIRI COCKTAIL MIX:**		
(Bacardi) frozen:		
Peach	4 fl.oz.	98
Raspberry	4 fl.oz.	97
Strawberry	4 fl.oz.	102
(Bar-Tender's)	3½ fl. oz.	177
(Holland House):		
Instant	.56 oz.	65
Liquid:		
Regular	1 oz.	36
Strawberry	1 oz.	31
DAIRY CRISP, cereal (Pet)	¼ cup	120
DAIRY QUEEN/BRAZIER:		
Banana split	13.5-oz. serving	540
Brownie Delight, hot fudge	9.4-oz. serving	600
Buster Bar	5¼-oz. piece	460
Chicken sandwich	7.8-oz. sandwich	670
Cone:		
Plain, any flavor, regular	5-oz. cone	240
Dipped, chocolate, regular	5½-oz. cone	340
Dilly Bar	3-oz. piece	210
Double Delight	9-oz. serving	490
DQ Sandwich	2.1-oz. sandwich	140
Fish sandwich:		
Plain	6-oz. sandwich	400
With cheese	6¼-oz. sandwich	440
Float	14-oz. serving	410
Freeze, vanilla	12-oz. serving	500
French fries:		
Regular	2½-oz. serving	200
Large	4-oz. serving	320
Frozen dessert	4-oz. serving	180
Hamburger:		
Plain:		
Single	5.2-oz. serving	360
Double	7.4-oz. serving	530

Food and Description	Measure or Quantity	Calories
Triple	9.6-oz. serving	710
With cheese:		
Single	5.7-oz. serving	410
Double	8.4-oz. serving	650
Triple	10.63-oz. serving	820
Hot dog:		
Regular:		
Plain	3.5-oz. serving	280
With cheese	4-oz. serving	330
With chili	4½-oz. serving	320
Super:		
Plain	6.2-oz. serving	520
With cheese	6.9-oz. serving	580
With chili	7.7-oz. serving	570
Malt, chocolate:		
Large	20¾-oz. serving	1060
Regular	14¾-oz. serving	760
Small	10¼-oz. serving	520
Mr. Misty:		
Plain:		
Large	15½-oz. serving	340
Regular	11.64-oz. serving	250
Small	8¼-oz. serving	190
Kiss	3.14-oz. serving	70
Float	14.5-oz. serving	390
Freeze	14.5-oz. serving	500
Onion rings	3-oz. serving	280
Parfait	10-oz. serving	430
Peanut Butter Parfait	10¾-oz. serving	750
Shake, chocolate:		
Large	20¾-oz. serving	990
Regular	14¾-oz. serving	710
Small	10¼-oz. serving	490
Strawberry shortcake	11-oz. serving	540
Sundae, chocolate:		
Large	8¾-oz. serving	440
Regular	6¼-oz. serving	310
Small	3¾-oz. serving	190
Tomato	½ oz.	4
DATE (Dromedary):		
Chopped	¼ cup	130
Pitted	5 dates	100
DE CHAUNAC WINE		
(Great Western) 12% alcohol	3 fl. oz.	71
DELI'S, frozen (Pepperidge Farm):		
Mexican style	4-oz. piece	280
Reuben in rye pastry	4-oz. piece	360

Food and Description	Measure or Quantity	Calories
Turkey, ham & cheese	4-oz. piece	270
DENNY'S RESTAURANT:		
BLT	1 order	542
Chef salad	1 order	263
Chicken:		
Sandwich, breast	1 sandwich	830
Steak, fried	1 order	606
Club sandwich	1 sandwich	614
Denny Burger	1 burger	537
Eggs, omelet, made with *Egg Beaters*	1 serving	225
Patty melt	1 serving	657
Super Bird	1 serving	600
Turkey sandwich, sliced	1 sandwich	445
DILL SEED (French's)	1 tsp.	9
DINERSAURS, cereal (Ralston Purina)	1 cup	110
DINNER, frozen (See individual listings such as BEEF; CHICKEN; TURKEY; etc.)		
DIP:		
Acapulco (Ortega) with cheddar cheese	1 oz.	64
Avocado (Nalley's)	1 oz.	114
Bacon & horseradish (Kraft)	1 T.	30
Bacon & onion (Nalley's)	1 oz.	113
Barbecue (Nalley's)	1 oz.	114
Bean (Eagle)	1 oz.	35
Blue cheese:		
(Dean) tangy	1 oz.	61
(Nalley's)	1 oz.	110
Chili (La Victoria)	1 T.	6
Chili bean (Old El Paso)	1 T.	8
Clam (Nalley's)	1 oz.	101
Cucumber (Kraft)	1 oz.	50
Cucumber & onion (Breakstone)	1 oz.	50
Guacamole (Calavo)	1 oz.	55
Hot bean (Hain)	1 T.	17
Jalapeño:		
Fritos	1 oz.	34
(Wise)	1 T.	12
Onion (Thank You Brand)	1 T.	45
Onion bean (Hain) natural	1 T.	17
Picante sauce (Wise)	1 T.	6
Taco (Hain)	1 T.	44
DIP 'UM SAUCE, canned (French's):		
BBQ	1 T.	22

Food and Description	Measure or Quantity	Calories
Hot mustard	1 T.	35
Sweet 'n sour	1 T.	40
DISTILLED LIQUOR, any brand:		
80 proof (40% alcohol)	1 fl. oz.	65
86 proof (43% alcohol)	1 fl. oz.	70
90 proof (45% alcohol)	1 fl. oz.	74
94 proof (47% alcohol)	1 fl. oz.	77
100 proof (50% alcohol)	1 fl. oz.	83
DOUGHNUT		
Regular:		
(Dolly Madison):		
Regular:		
Plain or coconut crunch	1¼-oz. piece	140
Chocolate coated	1¼-oz. piece	150
Dunkin' Stix	1⅜-oz. piece	210
Gems:		
Chocolate coated	.5-oz. piece	65
Powdered sugar	.5-oz. piece	10
Jumbo:		
Plain or cinnamon sugar	1.6-oz. piece	190
Sugar	1.7-oz. piece	210
Old fashioned:		
Chocolate glazed or powdered sugar	2.2-oz. piece	260
Cinnamon chip, glazed or orange crush	2.2-oz. piece	280
White iced	2.2-oz. piece	300
Dunkin' Donuts:		
Filled:		
Apple, with cinnamon sugar	1 piece	250
Bavarian, with chocolate frosting	1 piece	225
Blueberry	1 piece	240
Jelly	1 piece	220
Glazed:		
Buttermilk ring	1 piece	290
Chocolate ring	1 piece	324
French cruller	1 piece	140
Yeast ring	1 piece	200
Munchkin:		
Cake, with powdered sugar	1 piece	69
Chocolate, with glaze	1 piece	88
Plain cake ring	1 piece	270
(Hostess) Breakfast Bake Shop:		
Regular:		
Crumb, frosted	1¼-oz. piece	160
Glazed whirl	1 piece	190

Food and Description	Measure or Quantity	Calories
Honey wheat	1 piece	250
Old fashioned:		
Plain	1 piece	170
Glazed	1 piece	250
Donette Gems:		
Plain	1 piece	60
Cinnamon:		
Plain	1 piece	60
Apple filled	1 piece	70
Crumb, plain or frosted	1 piece	80
Powdered sugar, plain	1 piece	60
Family Pack:		
Cinnamon	1 piece	120
Powdered sugar	1 piece	120
Hostess O's:		
Plain	1 piece	230
Pantry	1 piece	190
(Hostess):		
Chocolate coated	1-oz. piece	130
Cinnamon	1-oz. piece	110
Donettes, powdered	1 piece	40
Old fashioned, plain	1.5-oz. piece	180
Powdered	1-oz. piece	110
Frozen (Morton):		
Regular:		
Boston creme	2-oz. piece	180
Chocolate iced	1.5-oz. piece	150
Jelly	1.8-oz. piece	180
Donut Holes	⅕ of 7¾-oz. pkg.	160
Morning Light, jelly	2.6-oz. piece	250
DRAMBUIE (Hiram Walker)	1 fl. oz.	110
DRUMSTICK, ice cream, frozen:		
Ice cream, in a cone:		
Topped with peanuts	1 piece	181
Topped with peanuts & cone bisque	1 piece	168
Ice milk, in a cone:		
Topped with peanuts	1 piece	163
Topped with peanuts & cone bisque	1 piece	150
DULCITO, frozen (Hormel) apple	4 oz.	290
DUMPLINGS, canned, dietetic (Dia-Mel)	8-oz. serving	160
DYNATRIM, mix, any flavor	1 serving	100

Food and Description	Measure or Quantity	Calories

E

ECLAIR:
Home recipe, with custard filling
  and chocolate icing | 4-oz. piece | 271
Frozen:
  (Rich's) chocolate | 2-oz. piece | 200
  (Weight Watchers) chocolate | 2.1-oz. piece | 120
EEL, smoked, meat only | 4 oz. | 374
EGG BREAKFAST, frozen:
(Aunt Jemima) homestyle, scrambled with hash browns | 5.7-oz. meal | 290
(Downyflake) scrambled:
  With ham & hash browns | 6¼-oz. meal | 360
  With hash browns & sausage | 6¼-oz. meal | 420
  With pecan twirl | 6¼-oz. meal | 510
(Swanson) *Great Starts*:
  Omelet, with cheese & ham | 7-oz. meal | 390
  Scrambled:
    & bacon, with home fries | 5.6-oz. meal | 340
    With cheese & cinnamon
      pancakes | 3.4-oz. meal | 290
    & home fries | 4.6-oz. meal | 260
    With mini oat bran muffins, reduced cholesterol | 4¾-oz. meal | 250
    & sausages, with hash browns | 6½-oz. meal | 430
EGG BREAKFAST, Sandwich, frozen:
(Swanson) *Great Starts*:
  On a biscuit:
    Canadian bacon & cheese | 5.2-oz. sandwich | 420
    Sausgae & cheese | 5½-oz. sandwich | 460
  On a muffin:
    Beefsteak & cheese | 4.9-oz. sandwich | 360
    Canadian bacon & cheese | 4.1-oz. sandwich | 290
(Weight Watchers) on an English
  muffin | 4-oz. sandwich | 230
EGG, CHICKEN:
Raw:
  White only | 1 large egg | 17
  Yolk only | 1 large egg | 59

Food and Description	Measure or Quantity	Calories
Boiled	1 large egg	81
Fried in butter	1 large egg	99
Omelet, mixed with milk & cooked in fat	1 large egg	107
Poached	1 large egg	78
Scrambled, mixed with milk & cooked in fat	1 large egg	111
*EGG FOO YUNG, dinner:		
(Chun King) stir fry	5 oz.	138
(La Choy)	1 patty plus ¼ cup sauce	164
EGG MIX (Durkee):		
Omelet:		
*With bacon	½ pkg.	310
*Puffy	½ pkg.	302
Scrambled:		
Plain	.8-oz. pkg.	124
With bacon	1.3-oz. pkg.	181
EGG NOG, dairy:		
(Borden)	½ cup	160
(Johanna Farms)	½ cup	195
EGG NOG COCKTAIL		
(Mr. Boston) 15% alcohol	3 fl. oz.	177
EGGPLANT:		
Boiled, drained	4 oz.	22
Frozen:		
(Buitoni) parmigiana	5 oz.	168
(Celentano) rollettes	11-oz. pkg.	320
(Mrs. Paul's) parmesan	5-oz. serving	240
(Weight Watchers) Parmesan	13-oz. pkg.	285
EGG ROLL, frozen:		
(Chun King):		
Chicken	3.6-oz. piece	220
Meat & shrimp	3.6-oz. piece	220
Shrimp	3.6-oz. piece	208
(La Choy):		
Almond chicken, entree	2 egg rolls	450
Beef & broccoli, entree	2 egg rolls	380
Chicken	.5-oz. piece	30
Lobster	3-oz. piece	180
Shrimp	.5-oz. piece	27
EGG ROLL DINNER, frozen		
(Van de Kamp's) Cantonese	10½-oz. serving	560
EGG ROLL WRAP (Nasoya)	1 piece	20
EGG SUBSTITUTE:		
Egg Magic (Featherweight)	½ envelope	60
*Scramblers (Morningstar Farms)	1 egg substitute	35

Food and Description	Measure or Quantity	Calories
Second Nature (Avoset)	3 T.	42
EL POLLO LOCO RESTAURANT:		
Beans	3½-oz. serving	110
Chicken	2 pieces (4.8-oz. edible portion)	310
Coleslaw	2.8-oz. serving	80
Combo meal	16-oz. serving	720
Corn	3.3-oz. serving	110
Dole Whip	4½-oz. serving	90
Potato salad	4.3-oz. serving	140
Rice	2½-oz. serving	100
Salsa	1.8-oz. serving	10
Tortilla:		
Corn	3.3-oz. serving	210
Flour	3.3-oz. serving	280
ENCHILADA OR ENCHILADA DINNER, frozen:		
Beef:		
(Banquet):		
Dinner	12-oz. meal	500
Entree	2-lb. pkg	1080
(Fred's) *Marquez*	7½-oz. serving	304
(Old El Paso)	11-oz. dinner	390
(Patio)	13¼-oz. meal	520
(Stouffer's) & bean, *Lean Cuisine*	9¼-oz. meal	280
(Swanson) 4-compartment dinner	13¾ oz. meal	480
(Van de Kamp's):		
Dinner, regular	12-oz. dinner	390
Entree, shredded	5½-oz. serving	180
(Weight Watchers) *Ultimate 200*, ranchero	9.1-oz. meal	190
Cheese:		
(Banquet)	12-oz. dinner	550
(Old El Paso) festive	11-oz. dinner	590
(Patio)	12¼-oz. meal	380
(Van de Kamp's)	12-oz. dinner	450
(Weight Watchers) ranchero	8.9-oz. meal	360
Chicken:		
(Old El Paso):		
Dinner, festive	11-oz. dinner	460
Entree, regular	1 piece	220
(Weight Watchers) suiza	9.4-oz. meal	330
ENCHILADA SAUCE:		
Canned:		
(El Molino) hot	1 T.	8
(La Victoria)	1 T.	5
(Old El Paso) hot	¼ cup	27

Food and Description	Measure or Quantity	Calories
*Mix (Durkee)	½ cup	29
ENCHILADA SEASONING MIX (Lawry's)	1.6-oz. pkg.	152
ENDIVE, CURLY OR ESCAROLE, cut	½ cup	7
ESPRESSO COFFEE LIQUEUR	1 fl. oz.	104

Food and Description	Measure or Quantity	Calories

F

Food and Description	Measure or Quantity	Calories
FAJITA, frozen:		
(Healthy Choice) beef	7-oz. meal	210
(Weight Watchers) chicken	6¾-oz. meal	230
FAJITA SEASONING MIX		
(Lawry's)	1.3-oz. pkg.	63
FARINA:		
(Hi-O) dry, regular	1 T.	46
(Malt-O-Meal) dry:		
Regular	1 oz.	96
Quick cooking	1 oz.	100
*(Pillsbury) made with water and salt	⅔ cup	80
FAT, COOKING:		
Crisco:		
Regular	1 T.	110
Butter flavor	1 T.	108
(Nu Made)	1 T.	110
(Rokeach) neutral nyafat	1 T.	99
Spry	1 T.	94
FENNEL SEED (French's)	1 tsp.	8
FETTUCINI, frozen:		
(Armour) *Dining Lite,* & broccoli	9-oz. meal	290
(Green Giant) primavera	9½-oz. meal	230
(Healthy Choice):		
Alfredo	8-oz. meal	270
Chickent	8½-oz. meal	240
(Stouffer's)	½ of 10-oz. pkg.	270
FIBER ONE, cereal (General Mills)	½ cup	60
FIG:		
Fresh	1½" fig	30
Canned, regular pack (Del Monte) whole, solids & liq.	½ cup	100
Dried (Sun-Maid), Calimyrna	½ cup	250
FIG JUICE (Sunsweet)	6 fl. oz.	120
FIGURINES (Pillsbury) all flavors	1 bar	100
FILBERT:		
Shelled	1 oz.	180

Food and Description	Measure or Quantity	Calories
(Fisher) oil dipped, salted	½ cup	360
FISH AND SHELLFISH, fresh, frozen and canned (See specific names: HADDOCK; OYSTER; etc.)		
***FISH BOUILLON** (Knorr)	8 fl.oz.	10
FISH CAKE, frozen:		
(Captain's Choice)	2-oz. piece	130
(Mrs. Paul's)	1 piece	95
FISH & CHIPS, frozen:		
(Gorton's)	1 pkg.	1350
(Swanson):		
Regular	10-oz. dinner	500
Homestyle Recipe	6½-oz. entree	340
FISH DINNER, frozen:		
(Banquet) platter	8-oz. dinner	270
(Gorton's) fillet in herb butter	1 pkg.	190
(Healthy Choice) lemon pepper	10.7-oz. meal	300
(Kid Cuisine) nuggets	7-oz. meal	320
(Morton)	9¾-oz. dinner	370
(Mrs. Paul's):		
Dijon	8¾ oz. entree	200
Mornay	9-oz. entree	230
(Stouffer's) *Lean Cuisine* filet, divan	10⅜-oz. meal	210
(Weight Watchers) *Ultimate 200*, oven baked	6.6-oz. meal	120
FISH FILLET, frozen:		
(Captain's Choice) fried, battered	3-oz. piece	240
(Frionor) *Bunch O' Crunch*, breaded	1 piece	140
(Gorton's):		
Regular, crunchy	1 piece	160
Light Recipe, tempura batter	1 piece	190
(Mrs. Paul's):		
Batter dipped	1 fillet	165
Crunchy batter	1 fillet	140
FISH KABOBS, frozen:		
(Mrs. Paul's) light batter	⅓ pkg.	200
(Van de Kamp's) batter dipped, french fried	4-oz. piece	240
FISH NUGGET, frozen (Frionor) *Bunch O' Crunch,* breaded	1 piece	40
FISH SANDWICH, frozen (Frionor) *Bunch O' Crunch,* microwave	5-oz. sandwich	320
FISH SEASONING (Featherweight)	¼ tsp.	1

Food and Description	Measure or Quantity	Calories
FISH STICKS, frozen:		
(Captain's Choice)	1 piece	76
(Frionor) *Bunch O' Crunch,*		
breaded	.7-oz. piece	58
(Gorton's) potato crisp	1 piece	65
(Mrs. Paul's):		
Batter fried	1 piece	52
Breaded & fried, crispy	1 piece	35
FIT'N FROSTY (Alba '77):		
Chocolate or marshmallow	1 envelope	70
Strawberry	1 envelope	74
Vanilla	1 envelope	69
FLOUNDER:		
Baked	4 oz.	229
Frozen:		
(Captain's Choice) fillet	3 oz.	99
(Frionor) *Norway Gourmet*	4-oz. fillet	60
(Gorton's) *Fishmarket Fresh*	5 oz.	110
FLOUNDER DINNER OR		
ENTREE, frozen:		
(Gorton's) stuffed, microwave		
entree	1 pkg.	350
(Mrs. Paul's) light	1 fillet	240
FLOUR:		
(Aunt Jemima) self-rising	¼ cup	109
Ballard, self-rising	¼ cup	100
Bisquick (Betty Crocker)	¼ cup	120
(Elam's):		
Brown rice, whole grain	¼ cup	146
Buckwheat, pure	¼ cup	92
Pastry	1 oz.	102
Rye, whole grain	¼ cup	89
Soy	1 oz.	98
Gold Medal (Betty Crocker)		
all-purpose or high protein	¼ cup	100
La Pina	¼ cup	100
(Mrs. Wright's) all-purpose, self-ris-		
ing or wheat	¼ cup	100
Pillsbury's Best:		
All-purpose or rye, medium	¼ cup	100
Sauce & gravy	2 T.	50
Self-rising	¼ cup	95
Presto, self-rising	¼ cup	98
Wondra	¼ cup	100
FOOD STICKS (Pillsbury) chocolate	1 piece	45
FRANKEN*BERRY, cereal		
(General Mills)	1 cup	110

Food and Description	Measure or Quantity	Calories
FRANKFURTER:		
(Eckrich):		
Beef or meat	1.6-oz. frankfurter	150
Beef or meat, jumbo	2-oz. frankfurter	190
Meat	1.2-oz. frankfurter	120
(Empire Kosher):		
Chicken	2-oz. frankfurter	106
Turkey	2-oz. frankfurter	107
(Healthy Choice) regular	1 frankfurter	50
Hebrew National:		
Beef	1.7-oz. frankfurter	149
Natural casing	2-oz. frankfurter	175
(Hormel):		
Beef	1.6-oz. frankfurter	139
Range Brand, Wrangler, smoked	1 frankfurter	160
(Hygrade) beef, *Ball Park*	2-oz. frankfurter	169
(Louis Rich) turkey	1.5-oz. frankfurter	95
(Morrison & Schiff)	1.7-oz. frankfurter	149
(Ohse):		
Regular, beef	1-oz. frankfurter	85
Wiener:		
Regular	1-oz. frankfurter	90
Chicken	1-oz. frankfurter	85
(Oscar Mayer):		
Bacon & cheddar	1.6-oz. frankfurter	139
Beef	1.6-oz. frankfurter	143
Cheese	1.6-oz. frankfurter	144
Little Wiener	2" frankfurter	28
Wiener	1.6-oz. frankfurter	144
(Perdue) chicken	1 oz.	71
(Safeway) premium, beef or meat	2-oz. frankfurter	170
(Smok-A-Roma) Beef	2-oz. frankfurter	170
FRENCH TOAST, frozen:		
(Aunt Jemima):		
Regular	1 slice	85
Cinnamon swirl	1 slice	97
(Downyflake):		
Plain	1 slice	135
Cinnamon	1 slice	105
Texas style, & sausage	4¼-oz. pkg.	400
(Swanson) *Great Starts*:		
Cinnamon swirl, with sausage	5½-oz.pkg.	390
Oatmeal, with lite links	4.6 oz. pkg.	310
(Weight Watchers):		
Cinnamon	3-oz. serving	160
With links	4½-oz. serving	270

Food and Description	Measure or Quantity	Calories
FRITTERS, frozen (Mrs. Paul's)		
apple or corn	2-oz. piece	120
FROOT LOOPS, cereal (Kellogg's)	1 cup	110
FROSTED RICE, cereal (Kellogg's)	1 cup	110
FROSTEE (Borden):		
Chocolate	1 cup	200
Strawberry	1 cup	180
FROSTS (Libby's):		
Dry:		
Banana	.5 oz.	50
Orange, strawberry or pineapple	.5 oz.	60
Liquid:		
Banana	7 fl. oz.	120
Orange or strawberry	8 fl. oz.	120
FROZEN DESSERT, dietetic (See also *TOFUTTI*):		
Regular:		
(Edy's):		
Chocolate	½ cup	140
Marble fudge	½ cup	160
Vanilla	½ cup	130
(Healthy Choice):		
Bordeaux cherry, neopolitan, strawberry or vanilla	4 oz.	120
Chocolate, cookies & cream or praline & caramel	4 oz.	130
Rocky Road	4 oz.	160
(Simplesse) *Simple Pleasures*:		
Original:		
Chocolate or pecan praline	½ cup	140
Chocolate chip	½ cup	150
Peach, strawberry or vanilla	½ cup	120
Light:		
Chocolate or vanilla	4 oz.	80
Vanilla fudge	4 oz.	90
(Weight Watchers):		
Bulk, fat free:		
Chocolate, neopolitan or vanilla	½ cup	80
Chocolate swirl	½ cup	90
Bar, chocolate mousse, sugar free	1 bar	35
Non-dairy:		
(Carnation) *Lite Wonder*:		
Chocolate or strawberry	½ cup	110
Mocha fudge	½ cup	120

Food and Description	Measure or Quantity	Calories
Mocha Mix (Presto Food):		
Chocolate chip	4 oz.	180
Dutch chocolate or neopolitan	4 oz.	130
Toasted almond	4 oz.	150
(Sealtest) Free, any flavor	½ cup	100
FRUIT, MIXED:		
Canned (Del Monte) lite, chunky	½ cup	58
Dried (Twon House)	2 oz.	150
Frozen (Birds Eye) quick thaw	5-oz. serving	150
FRUIT BARS (General Mills) *Fruit Corners*	1 bar	90
FRUIT BITS, dried (Sun-Maid)	1 oz.	90
FRUIT COCKTAIL:		
Canned, regular pack, solids & liq.:		
(Hunt's)	4 oz.	90
(Libby's)	½ cup	101
(Stokely-Van Camp)	½ cup	95
(Town House)	½ cup	90
Canned, dietetic or low calorie, solids & liq.:		
(Country Pure) Lite	½ cup	50
(Diet Delight):		
Syrup pack	½ cup	50
Water pack	½ cup	40
(Featherweight):		
Juice pack	½ cup	50
Water pack	½ cup	40
(Libby's) water pack	½ cup	50
(S&W) *Nutradiet:*		
Juice pack	½ cup	50
Water pack	½ cup	40
FRUIT COMPOTE (Rokeach)	½ cup	120
FRUIT COUNTRY (Comstock):		
Apple or blueberry	¼ pkg.	160
Cherry	¼ pkg.	180
FRUIT & CREAM BAR (Dole):		
Blueberry, peach or strawberry	1 bar	90
Chocolate-banana	1 bar	175
Chocolate-strawberry	1 bar	160
FRUIT CUP (Del Monte):		
Mixed fruits	5-oz. container	110
Peaches, diced	5-oz. container	116
FRUIT & FIBRE CEREAL (Post):		
Dates, raisins, walnuts with oat clusters	⅔ cup	120
Tropical fruit with oat clusters	⅔ cup	125
FRUIT JUICE, canned (Sun-Maid)	6 fl. oz.	100

Food and Description	Measure or Quantity	Calories
FRUIT 'N APPLE JUICE (Tree Top)	6 fl. oz.	90
FRUIT 'N GRAPE JUICE (Tree Top):		
Canned	6 fl. oz.	100
*Frozen	6 fl. oz.	110
FRUIT & JUICE BAR:		
(Dole):		
Regular:		
Cherry, peach, passion fruit or pineapple	1 bar	70
Piña colada	1 bar	80
Raspberry or strawberry	1 bar	60
Fresh lites, any flavor	1 bar	25
Sun Tops	1 bar	40
(Weight Watchers)	1 bar	35
FRUIT & NUT MIX (Carnation):		
All fruit	.9-oz. pouch	80
Deluxe trail mix or raisins & nuts	.9-oz. pouch	130
Tropical fruit & nuts	.9-oz. pouch	100
FRUIT PUNCH:		
Canned:		
Capri Sun	6¾ fl. oz.	102
(Hi-C)	6 fl. oz.	96
(Lincoln)	6 fl. oz.	90
(Minute Maid):		
Regular	8.45-fl.-oz. container	128
On the Go	10-fl.-oz. bottle	152
Chilled:		
(Minute Maid)	6 fl.oz.	91
(Sunkist)	8.45 fl. oz.	140
*Frozen, *Five Alive* (Snow Crop)	6 fl. oz.	87
FRUIT RINGS, cereal (Safeway)	1 oz.	110
FRUIT ROLL:		
(Flavor Tree)	⅜-oz. roll	80
Fruit Roll-Ups, Fruit Corners	.5-oz. roll	50
FRUIT SALAD:		
Canned, regular pack:		
(Dole) tropical	½ cup	70
(Libby's)	½ cup	99
Canned, dietetic or low calorie:		
(Diet Delight)	½ cup	60
(Featherweight):		
Juice pack	½ cup	50
Water pack	½ cup	40

Food and Description	Measure or Quantity	Calories
(S&W) *Nutradiet:*		
Juice pack	½ cup	60
Water pack	½ cup	35
FRUIT SLUSH (Wyler's)	4 fl.oz.	157
FRUIT WRINKLES (General Mills)		
Fruit Corners	1 pouch	100
FRUITY YUMMY MUMMY, cereal		
(General Mills)	1 cup (1 oz.)	110
FUDGSICLE (Popsicle Industries)	2½-fl.-oz. bar	100

Food and Description	Measure or Quantity	Calories

G

GARFIELD AND FRIENDS
(General Mills):
  Pouch:

1-2 Punch	.9-oz. pouch	100
Very strawberry	.9-oz. pouch	90
Roll	.5-oz. roll	50

GARLIC:

Flakes (Gilroy)	1 tsp.	5
Powder (French's) with parsley	1 tsp.	12
Salt (Lawry's)	1 tsp.	4
Spread (Lawry's) concentrate	1 T.	15
GATORADE, canned, Fruit punch, lemon-lime, or orange	8 fl. oz.	50

GEFILTE FISH, canned:
  (Manischewitz):

Fishlets	1 piece	8
Gefilte:		
Regular:		
12 or 24-oz. container	1 piece (3 oz.)	53
4-lb. container	1 piece (2.7 oz.)	48
Homestyle, 12 or 24-oz. container	1 piece (3 oz.)	55
Sweet, 12 or 24-oz. container	1 piece (3 oz.)	65
Whitefish & pike:		
Regular, 12 or 24-oz. container	1 piece (3 oz.)	49
Sweet, 4-lb. container	1 piece (2.7 oz.)	58
(Mother's):		
Jellied, Old World	4-oz. serving	70
Jellied, white fish & pike	4-oz. serving	60
In liquid broth	4-oz. serving	70
(Rokeach):		
Natural Broth	2-oz. serving	46
Old Vienna:		
Regular	2-oz. serving	52
Jelled	2-oz. serving	54
GELATIN, dry, *Carmel Kosher*	7-gram envelope	30

*GELATIN DESSERT MIX:
  Regular:

Carmel Kosher, all flavors	½ cup	80

Food and Description	Measure or Quantity	Calories
(Jell-O) all flavors	½ cup	81
(Jell-Well) all flavors	½ cup	80
Dietetic:		
Carmel Kosher	½ cup	8
(D-Zerta) all flavors	½ cup	6
(Featherweight) artificially sweetened or regular	½ cup	10
(Jell-Well) all flavors	½ cup	8
*(Royal)	½ cup	12
GELATIN, DRINKING (Knox) orange	1 envelope	39
GERMAN-STYLE DINNER, frozen (Swanson)	11⅜-oz. dinner	370
GIN, SLOE:		
(Bols)	1 fl. oz.	85
(DeKuyper)	1 fl. oz.	70
(Mr. Boston)	1 fl. oz.	68
GINGER, powder (French's)	1 tsp.	6
GINGERBREAD:		
Home recipe (USDA)	1.9-oz. piece	174
Mix:		
*(Betty Crocker):		
Regular	⅑ of pkg.	220
No cholesterol recipe	⅑ of pkg.	210
(Dromedary)	2" × 2" square	100
(Pillsbury)	3" square	190
GOLDEN GRAHAMS, cereal (General Mills)	¾ cup	110
GOOBER GRAPE (Smucker's)	1 T.	90
GOOD HUMOR (See ICE CREAM)		
GOOD N' PUDDIN (Popsicle Industries) all flavors	2⅓-fl.-oz. bar	170
GOOSE, roasted, meat & skin	4 oz.	500
GRAHAM CRAKOS, cereal (Kellogg's)	1 cup	110
GRANOLA BAR:		
(Health Valley) fat free, blueberry apple, date almond, or raspberry	1 bar	140
(Hershey's) chocolate chip	1.2-oz. piece	170
(Nature Valley):		
Chocolate chip or oat bran honey graham	1 bar	110
Cinnamon or peanut butter	1 bar	120
Rice bran-cinnamon raisin	1 bar	90

Food and Description	Measure or Quantity	Calories
(Nature's Choice)	1 bar	90
(Ultra Slim Fast) nutrition, any flavor	1 bar	140
GRANOLA CEREAL:		
Nature Valley:		
Cinnamon & raisin, fruit & nut or toasted oat	⅓ cup	130
Coconut & honey	⅓ cup	150
Sun Country:		
With almonds	1 oz.	130
With raisins & dates	1 oz.	130
GRANOLA CLUSTERS,		
Nature Valley:		
Almond	1 piece	140
Caramel & raisin	1 piece	150
GRANOLA & FRUIT BAR,		
Nature Valley	1 bar	150
GRANOLA SNACK:		
Kudos (M&M/Mars):		
Chocolate chip	1.25-oz. pkg.	180
Peanut butter	1.3-oz. pkg.	190
Nature Valley	1 pouch	140
GRAPE:		
American, ripe (slipskin)	3½" × 3" bunch	43
Canned, dietetic (Featherweight) light, seedless, water pack	½ cup	60
GRAPEADE: (Minute Maid) chilled or *frozen	6 fl.oz.	94
GRAPE-APPLE DRINK, canned (Mott's)	6 fl.oz.	100
GRAPE DRINK:		
Canned:		
Bama (Borden)	8.45-fl.-oz.	120
(Hi-C)	6 fl. oz.	96
(Johanna Farms) *Ssips*	8.45-fl.-oz.	130
(Lincoln)	6 fl. oz.	90
Chilled (Sunkist)	8.45-fl.-oz.	140
*Mix:		
Regular (Funny Face)	6 fl. oz.	66
Dietetic (Sunkist)	8 fl. oz.	6
GRAPE JAM (Smucker's)	1 T.	53
GRAPE JELLY:		
Sweetened:		
Bama (Borden)	1 T.	45
(Smucker's)	1 T.	53
(Welch's)	1 T.	52

Food and Description	Measure or Quantity	Calories
Dietetic:		
(Diet Delight)	1 T.	12
(Estee)	1 T.	6
(Welch's)	1 T.	30
GRAPE JUICE:		
Canned, unsweetened:		
(Ardmore Farms)	6 fl. oz.	99
(Johanna Farms) *Tree Ripe*	8.45-fl.-oz.	164
(Minute Maid)	8.45-fl.-oz. container	150
(Seneca Foods)	6 fl. oz.	118
(Town House)	6 fl. oz.	70
(Tree Top) sparkling	6 fl. oz.	120
(Welch's) regular or red	6 fl. oz.	120
Chilled (Minute Maid)	6 fl. oz.	100
*Frozen:		
(Bel-Air)	6 fl. oz.	200
(Minute Maid)	6 fl. oz.	100
(Welch's)	6 fl. oz.	100
*GRAPE JUICE DRINK, frozen		
(Sunkist)	6 fl. oz.	69
GRAPEFRUIT:		
Pink & red:		
Seeded type	½ med. grapefruit	46
Seedless type	½ med. grapefruit	49
White:		
Seeded type	½ med. grapefruit	44
Seedless type	½ med. grapefruit	46
Canned, regular pack (Del Monte) in syrup	½ cup	74
Canned, dietetic pack, solids & liq.:		
(Del Monte) sections	½ cup	45
(Diet Delight) sections	½ cup	45
(Featherweight) sections, juice pack	½ cup	40
(S&W) *Nutradiet*	½ cup	40
GRAPEFRUIT DRINK, canned		
(Lincoln)	6 fl. oz.	104
GRAPEFRUIT JUICE:		
Fresh, pink, red or white	½ cup	46
Canned, sweetened:		
(Ardmore Farms)	6 fl. oz.	78
(Libby's)	6 fl. oz.	70
(Minute Maid) On the Go	10-fl.-oz. bottle	130
(Mott's)	10-fl.oz. container	124
(Texsun)	6 fl. oz.	77
Canned, unsweetened:		

Food and Description	Measure or Quantity	Calories
(Ocean Spray)	6 fl. oz.	70
(Texsun)	6 fl. oz.	77
(Town House)	6 fl. oz.	120
(Tree Top)	6 fl. oz.	80
Chilled (Sunkist)	6 fl. oz.	72
*Frozen:		
(A&P)	6 fl. oz.	80
(Minute Maid)	6 fl.oz.	83
(Sunkist)	6 fl.oz.	56
GRAPEFRUIT JUICE COCKTAIL,		
canned (Ocean Spray) pink	6 fl. oz.	80
GRAPE NUTS, cereal (Post)	¼ cup (1 oz.)	105
GRAVY, canned:		
Au jus (Franco-American)	2-oz. serving	10
Beef (Franco-American)	2-oz. serving	25
Brown:		
(Estee) dietetic	¼ cup	14
(Heinz) plain or with onions, home style	2-oz. serving	25
(La Choy)	2 oz.	140
Ready Gravy	¼ cup	44
Chicken (Franco-American):		
Regular	2-oz. serving	45
Giblet	2-oz. serving	30
Chicken & herb	¼ cup	20
Cream (Franco-American)	2 oz.	35
Mushroom (Franco-American)	2 oz. serving	25
Pork (Franco-American)	2 oz. serving	40
Turkey:		
(Franco-American)	2 oz. serving	30
(Howard Johnson's) giblet	½ cup	55
GRAVYMASTER	1 tsp.	11
*GRAVY MIX:		
Regular:		
Au jus:		
(Durkee)	½ cup	15
(French's) *Gravy Makins*	½ cup	20
Brown:		
(Durkee) regular	½ cup	29
(French's) *Gravy Makins*	½ cup	40
(Knorr) classic	2 fl. oz.	25
(Lawry's)	½ cup	47
(Pillsbury)	½ cup	30
(Spatini)	1 oz.	8
Chicken:		
(Durkee) regular	½ cup	43
(French's) *Gravy Makins*	½ cup	50

Food and Description	Measure or Quantity	Calories
(Pillsbury)	½ cup	50
Home style:		
(Durkee)	½ cup	35
(French's) *Gravy Makins*	½ cup	40
(Pillsbury)	½ cup	30
Meatloaf (Durkee) *Roasting Bag*	1.5-oz. pkg.	129
Mushroom:		
(Durkee)	½ cup	30
(French's) *Gravy Makins*	½ cup	40
Onion:		
(Durkee)	½ cup	42
(French's) *Gravy Makins*	½ cup	50
(McCormick)	.85-oz. pkg.	72
Pork:		
(Durkee)	½ cup	35
(French's) *Gravy Makins*	½ cup	40
Swiss Steak (Durkee)	½ cup	23
Turkey:		
(Durkee)	½ cup	47
(French's) *Gravy Makins*	½ cup	50
Dietetic (Estee):		
Brown	½ cup	28
Chicken	½ cup	40
GRAVY WITH MEAT OR TURKEY, frozen:		
(Banquet):		
Cookin' Bag:		
Mushroom gravy & charbroiled beef patty	5-oz. pkg.	210
& salisbury steak	5-oz. pkg.	190
& sliced turkey	5-oz. pkg.	100
Family Entree:		
Onion gravy & beef patties	¼ of 32-oz. pkg.	300
& sliced beef	¼ of 32-oz. pkg.	160
(Swanson) sliced beef	8-oz. entree	200
GREAT BEGINNINGS		
(Hormel):		
With chunky beef	5 oz.	136
With chunky chicken	5 oz.	147
With chunky turkey	5 oz.	138
GREENS, MIXED, canned:		
(Allen's)	½ cup	25
(Sunshine) solids & liq.	½ cup	20
GRENADINE (Rose's) no alcohol	1 fl. oz.	65
GUACAMOLE SEASONING MIX		
(Lawry's)	.7-oz. pkg.	60

Food and Description	Measure or Quantity	Calories
GUAVA	1 guava	48
GUAVA FRUIT DRINK, canned,		
Mauna L'ai	6 fl. oz.	100
GUAVA NECTAR (Libby's)	6 fl. oz.	70

Food and Description	Measure or Quantity	Calories

H

HADDOCK:

Food and Description	Measure or Quantity	Calories
Fried, breaded	4" × 3" × ½" fillet	165
Frozen:		
(Captain's Choice) fillet	3 oz.	95
(Gorton's) *Fishmarket Fresh*	5-oz. piece	110
(Mrs. Paul's) fillet, light	1 piece	110
(Van de Kamp's) batter dipped, french fried	2-oz. piece	120
(Weight Watchers) with stuffing, 2-compartment	7-oz. pkg.	205
Smoked	4-oz. serving	117
HALIBUT:		
Broiled	4" × 3" × ½" steak	214
Frozen (Captain's Choice) steak	3 oz.	119
HAM:		
Canned:		
(Hormel):		
Black Label (3- or 5-lb. size)	4 oz.	140
Chunk	6¾-oz. serving	310
Patties	1 patty	180
(Oscar Mayer) *Jubilee,* extra lean, cooked	1-oz. serving	31
(Swift) *Premium*	1¾-oz. slice	111
Deviled:		
(Hormel)	1 T.	35
(Libby's)	1 T.	43
(Underwood)	1 T.	49
Packaged:		
(Carl Buddig) smoked	1 oz.	50
(Eckrich):		
Loaf	1 oz.	70
Cooked or imported, Danish	1.2-oz. slice	30
(Hormel):		
Black, or red peppered or frozen	1 slice	25
Chopped	1 slice	55
(Ohse):		
Chopped	1 oz.	65

Food and Description	Measure or Quantity	Calories
Cooked	1 oz.	30
Smoked, regular	1 oz.	45
(Oscar Mayer):		
Baked	.7-oz. slice	21
Black pepper	.7-oz. slice	22
Boiled	.7-oz. slice	23
Breakfast	1½-oz. slice	48
Chopped	1-oz. slice	52
Cooked, smoked	¾-oz. slice	22
Jubilee, boneless:		
Sliced	8-oz. slice	232
Steak, 95% fat free	2-oz. steak	58
(Smok-A-Roma) honey	1-oz. slice	30
HAM & ASPARAGUS BAKE,		
frozen (Stouffer's)	9½-oz. meal	510
HAM & CHEESE:		
(Eckrich) loaf	1-oz. serving	60
(Hormel) loaf	1-oz. serving	65
(Ohse) loaf	1 oz.	65
(Oscar Mayer)	1-oz. slice	66
HAM AND CHEESE		
BREAKFAST, on a bagel, frozen		
(Swanson) *Great Starts*	3-oz. pkg.	240
HAM DINNER, frozen:		
(Armour) *Dinner Classics,* steak	10⅜-oz. dinner	270
(Banquet) platter	10-oz. meal	400
(Le Menu) steak	10-oz. dinner	300
(Morton)	10-oz. dinner	290
HAM SALAD, canned (Carnation)	¼ of 7½-oz. can	110
HAM SALAD SPREAD		
(Oscar Mayer)	1 oz.	59
HAMBURGER (See *BURGER KING; DAIRY QUEEN; McDONALD'S; WHITE CASTLE;* etc. See also *BEEF,* ground)		
HAMBURGER MIX:		
Hamburger Helper (General Mills):		
Beef noodle or hamburger hash	⅕ pkg.	320
Cheeseburger macaroni	⅕ pkg.	370
Chili, with beans	¼ pkg.	350
Hamburger stew	⅕ pkg.	300
Lasagna	⅕ pkg.	340
Sloppy Joe Bake	⅕ pkg.	340

Food and Description	Measure or Quantity	Calories
Make a Better Burger (Lipton) mildly seasoned or onion	⅓ pkg.	30
HAMBURGER SEASONING MIX:		
*(Durkee)	1 cup	663
(French's)	1-oz. pkg.	100
HARDEE'S RESTAURANT:		
Apple turnover	3.2-oz. piece	270
Big Cookie	1.7-oz. piece	250
Big Country Breakfast:		
Bacon	7.65-oz. meal	660
Country ham	8.96-oz. meal	670
Ham	8.85-oz. meal	620
Sausage	9.7-oz. meal	850
Biscuit:		
Bacon	3.3-oz. serving	360
Bacon & egg	4.4-oz. serving	410
Bacon, egg & cheese	4.8-oz. serving	460
Chicken	5.1-oz. serving	430
Country ham:		
Plain	3.8-oz. serving	350
& egg	4.9-oz. serving	400
'n gravy	7.8-oz. serving	440
Ham:		
Plain	3.7-oz. serving	320
With egg	4.9-oz. serving	370
With egg & cheese	5.3-oz. serving	420
Rise 'N Shine:		
Plain	2.9-oz. serving	320
Canadian bacon	5.7-oz. serving	470
Sausage:		
Plain	4.2-oz. serving	440
With egg	5.3-oz. serving	490
Steak:		
Plain	5.2-oz. serving	500
With egg	6.3-oz. serving	550
Cheeseburger:		
Plain	4.3-oz. serving	320
Bacon	7.7-oz. serving	610
Quarter-pound	6.4-oz. serving	500
Chicken fillet sandwich	6.1-oz. sandwich	370
Chicken, grilled, sandwich	6.8-oz. sandwich	310
Chicken Stix:		
6-piece	3½-oz. serving	210
9-piece	5.3-oz. serving	310
Cool Twist:		
Cone:		
Chocolate	4.2-oz. serving	200

Food and Description	Measure or Quantity	Calories
Vanilla	4.2-oz. serving	190
Vanilla/chocolate	4.2-oz. serving	190
Sundae:		
Caramel	6-oz. serving	330
Hot fudge	5.9-oz. serving	320
Strawberry	5.9-oz. serving	260
Fisherman's Fillet, sandwich	7.3-oz. sandwich	500
Hamburger:		
Plain	3.9-oz. serving	270
Big Deluxe	7.6-oz. serving	500
Mushroom 'N Swiss	6.6-oz. serving	490
Hot dog, all beef	4.2-oz. serving	300
Hot ham 'n cheese	4.2-oz. sandwich	330
Margarine/butter blend	.2-oz. serving	35
Pancakes, three:		
Plain	4.8-oz. serving	280
With sausage pattie	6.2-oz. serving	430
With bacon strips	5.3-oz. serving	350
Potato:		
French fries:		
Regular	2½-oz. order	230
Large	4-oz. order	360
Hash Rounds	2.8-oz. serving	230
Roast beef:		
Regular	4-oz. serving	260
Big Roast Beef	4.7-oz. serving	300
Salads:		
Chef	10.4-oz. serving	240
Chicken & pasta	14.6-oz. serving	230
Garden	8.5-oz. serving	210
Side	3.9-oz. serving	20
Sauce:		
Barbecue dipping	1 oz.	30
Honey	.5 oz.	45
Sweet mustard dipping	1 oz.	50
Tartar	.7 oz.	90
Shake:		
Chocolate	12 fl. oz.	460
Strawberry	12 fl. oz.	440
Vanilla	12 fl. oz.	400
Syrup	1½-oz. serving	120
Turkey club sandwich	7.3-oz. serving	390
HEADCHEESE (Oscar Mayer)	1-oz. serving	55
HEARTWISE, cereal (Kellogg's)	⅔ cup (1 oz.)	90
HERRING, canned (Vita):		
Cocktail, drained	8-oz. jar	342
In cream sauce	8-oz. jar	397

Food and Description	Measure or Quantity	Calories
Tastee Bits, drained	8-oz. jar	361
HERRING, SMOKED, kippered	4-oz. serving	239
HICKORY NUT, shelled	1 oz.	191
HOMINY, canned (Allen's) golden, solids & liq.	½ cup	80
HOMINY GRITS:		
Dry:		
(Albers)	1½ oz.	150
(Aunt Jemima)	3 T.	102
(Quaker):		
Regular	3 T.	101
Instant:		
Regular	.8-oz. packet	79
With imitation bacon or ham	1-oz. packet	101
Cooked	1 cup	125
HONEY, strained	1 T.	61
HONEY BUNCHES OF OATS, cereal (Post):		
With almonds	⅔ cup (1 oz.)	115
Honey roasted	⅔ cup (1 oz.)	111
HONEYCOMB, cereal (Post) regular	1⅓ cups (1 oz.)	110
HONEYDEW	2" × 7" wedge	31
HONEY SMACKS, cereal (Kellogg's)	¾ cup (1 oz.)	110
HORSERADISH:		
Raw, pared	1 oz.	25
Prepared (Gold's)	1 tsp.	4
HOT BITES, frozen (Banquet):		
Cheese, mozzarella nuggets	¼ of 10½-oz. pkg.	240
Chicken:		
Regular:		
Breast patty, regular or southern fried	¼ of 10½-oz. pkg.	210
Drum snackers	¼ of 10½-oz. pkg.	220
Nuggets:		
Plain	¼ of 10½-oz. pkg.	210
With cheddar or hot & spicy	¼ of 10½-oz. pkg.	250
Southern fried	¼ of 10½-oz. pkg.	220
Microwave:		
Breast pattie:		
Regular, & bun	4-oz. pkg.	310
Southern fried, & biscuit	4-oz. pkg.	320
Nuggets, hot & spicy, with BBQ sauce	4½-oz. pkg.	360
HOT DOG (See FRANKFURTER)		
HOT WHEELS, cereal (Ralston Purina)	1 cup	110
HULA COOLER (Hi-C)	6 fl. oz.	97

Food and Description	Measure or Quantity	Calories

I

ICE CREAM (Listed by type, such as sandwich, or *Whammy,* or by flavor—See also FROZEN DESSERT):

Food and Description	Measure or Quantity	Calories
Almond (Good Humor) supreme	4 fl. oz.	350
Almond amaretto (Baskin-Robbins)	4 fl. oz.	280
Apple strudel (Lucerne)	½ cup	140
Banana crumble (Lucerne)	½ cup	140
Bar:		
(Dove Bar):		
Regular:		
Almond	1 bar	350
Chocolate:		
Dark chocolate coating	1 bar	350
Milk chocolate coating	1 bar	340
Vanilla, with dark or milk chocolate coating	1 bar	340
Light, vanilla with dark or milk chocolate coating	1 bar	230
(Good Humor):		
Chip candy crunch	3-fl.-oz. bar	255
Chocolate Eclair	3-fl.-oz. bar	187
Halo bar	2½-fl.-oz. bar	230
Shark bar	3-fl.-oz. bar	68
Strawberry shortcake	3-fl.-oz. bar	176
Toasted almond	3-fl.-oz. bar	212
Vanilla, chocolate coated	3-fl.-oz. bar	198
(Häagen-Dazs):		
Chocolate with dark chocolate coating	1 bar	360
Fudge	1 bar	210
Vanilla with milk chocolate coating	1 bar	320
(Lucerne) chocolate fudge	3-fl.-oz. bar	125
Blueberry & cream (Häagen-Dazs)	4 fl. oz.	190
Bon Bon (Carnation) vanilla	1 piece	33
Brittle bar (Häagen-Dazs)	1 bar	370
Brownie sundae (Lucerne)	½ cup	140

Food and Description	Measure or Quantity	Calories
Butter Almond (Breyers)	½ cup	170
Butter pecan:		
(Breyer's)	¼ pt.	180
(Häagen-Dazs)	4 fl. oz.	290
(Lady Borden)	½ cup	180
(Lucerne) gourmet	½ cup	190
Cappuccino (Baskin-Robbins) chip	4 fl. oz.	310
Chocolate:		
(Baskin-Robbins):		
Regular	4 fl. oz.	264
Mousse Royale	4 fl. oz.	293
(Borden) old fashioned recipe	½ cup	130
(Breyers)	½ cup	160
(Good Humor) bulk	4 fl. oz.	130
(Häagen-Dazs) mint	4 fl. oz.	300
(Lucerne):		
Regular	½ cup	140
Dietary	½ cup	130
(Snow Star)	½ cup	120
Chocolate fudge (Häagen-Dazs) deep	4 fl. oz.	300
Chocolate marshmallow (Lucerne)	½ cup	140
Chocolate peanut butter (Häagen-Dazs)	4 fl. oz.	330
Chocolate raspberry truffle (Baskin-Robbins)	4 fl. oz.	310
Chocolate swirl (Borden)	½ cup	130
Coconut almond fudge (Lucerne)	½ cup	150
Coffee:		
(Breyers)	½ cup	140
(Häagen-Dazs)	4 fl. oz.	270
(Lucerne)	½ cup	140
Cookies & cream:		
(Breyers)	½ cup	170
(Sealtest)	½ cup	150
Cookie sandwich (Good Humor)	2.7-fl.-oz. piece	290
Egg nog (Lucerne) gourmet	½ cup	160
Eskimo Pie, vanilla with chocolate coating	3-fl.-oz. bar	180
Eskimo, Thin Mint, with chocolate coating	2-fl.-oz. bar	140
Fat Frog (Good Humor)	3-fl.-oz. pop	154
Fudge cake (Good Humor)	6.3 fl. oz.	214
Fudge royal (Sealtest)	½ cup	140
Grand Marnier (Baskin-Robbins)	4 fl. oz.	240
Honey (Häagen-Dazs)	4 fl. oz.	250
Jamocha (Baskin-Robbins)	1 scoop (2½ fl. oz.)	146

Food and Description	Measure or Quantity	Calories
Jamocha almond fudge (Baskin-Robbins)	4 fl. oz.	270
Jumbo Jet Star (Good Humor)	4.5 fl. oz.	84
Key lime & cream (Häagen-Dazs)	4 fl. oz.	200
King cone (Good Humor) boysenberry	5 fl.oz.	340
Macadamia nut (Häagen-Dazs)	4 fl. oz.	280
Maple walnut (Häagen-Dazs)	4 fl. oz.	310
Milky pop (Good Humor)	1.5-fl.-oz. piece	46
Mocha double nut (Häagen-Dazs)	4 fl. oz.	290
Mocha fudge (Lucerne) nut	½ cup	150
Orange & cream (Häagen-Dazs)	4 fl. oz.	200
Oreo, Cookies 'n Cream:		
Bulk	3 fl. oz.	140
Sandwich	1 piece	240
Peach (Häagen-Dazs)	4 fl. oz.	212
Peanut butter (Lucerne) cup	½ cup	145
Pralines 'N Cream (Baskin-Robbins)	1 scoop (2½ fl. oz.)	177
Rocky Road (Baskin-Robbins)	4 fl. oz.	300
Rum raisin (Häagen-Dazs)	4 fl. oz.	250
Sandwich (Good Humor) vanilla	2½-oz. piece	161
Strawberry:		
(Baskin-Robbins) wild, light	4 fl. oz.	90
(Borden)	½ cup	130
(Häagen-Dazs)	4 fl. oz.	250
(Lucerne) regular	½ cup	130
(Snow Star)	½ cup	115
Strawberry & cream:		
(Borden) old fashioned recipe	½ cup	130
(Good Humor)	4 fl. oz.	94
Supreme (Good Humor) milk	4 fl. oz.	278
Tin Lizzy (Lucerne)	½ cup	140
Vanilla:		
(Baskin-Robbins) regular	4 fl. oz.	235
(Borden)	½ cup	130
(Eagle Brand)	½ cup	150
(Häagen-Dazs)	4 fl. oz.	260
(Land O' Lakes)	4 fl. oz.	140
(Lucerne):		
Regular	½ cup	140
French	½ cup	150
(Sealtest)	½ cup	140
(Snow Star)	½ cup	130
Vanilla caramel (Häagen-Dazs)	4 fl. oz.	310

Food and Description	Measure or Quantity	Calories
Vanilla & caramel triple nut (Häagen-Dazs)	4 fl. oz.	310
Vanilla-chocolate cup (Good Humor)	6 fl. oz.	201
Vanilla cup (Good Humor)	3 fl. oz.	98
Vanilla sandwich (Good Humor)	3 fl. oz.	191
Vanilla Swiss almond (Häagen-Dazs)	4 fl. oz.	290
Whammy (Good Humor) assorted	1.6-oz. piece	95
ICE CREAM CONE, cone only:		
(Baskin-Robbins):		
Sugar	1 cone	60
Waffle	1 cone	140
(Comet) sugar	1 cone	40
ICE CREAM CUP, cup only		
(Comet) regular	1 cup	20
***ICE CREAM MIX** (Salada)		
any flavor	1 cup	310
ICE MILK:		
Hardened	¼ pt.	100
Soft-serve	¼ pt.	133
(Borden):		
Chocolate	½ cup	100
Vanilla	½ cup	90
(Carnation) *Smooth 'N Lite*:		
Cherry vanilla	½ cup	100
Chocolate, strawberry, or vanilla	½ cup	90
Cookies & cream or rocky road	½ cup	120
Double dutch fudge or marble fudge	½ cup	150
Vanilla bean	½ cup	140
(Crystal Light) *Cool 'N Creamy*, bars:		
Bavarian, double chocolate fudge or orange	1 bar	50
Chocolate Amaretto	1 bar	60
(Land O' Lakes) vanilla	4 fl. oz.	110
(Light N' Lively):		
Caramel nut, chocolate chip or heavenly hash	½ cup	120
Vanilla	½ cup	100
Vanilla/chocolate/strawberry	½ cup	110
(Lucerne):		
Regular:		
Carmel nut	½ cup	105
Chocolate, regular or marble	½ cup	110

Food and Description	Measure or Quantity	Calories
Rocky road	½ cup	110
Vanilla	½ cup	100
Light:		
Chocolate	½ cup	120
Strawberry	½ cup	110
Toasted almond	½ cup	125
(Meadow Gold) vanilla, 4% fat	¼ pt.	95
(Sweet 'N Low) bar, vanilla with chocolate coating	1 bar	90
(Weight Watchers):		
Bars:		
Caramel nut or English toffee crunch	1 bar	120
Chocolate crispy treat or chocolate dip	1 bar	110
Bulk:		
Grand Collection:		
Chocolate or neapolitan	½ cup	110
Chocolate chip, chocolate swirl, or pecan praline & cream	½ cup	120
Vanilla	½ cup	100
One-Ders:		
Chocolate chip	½ cup	120
Heavenly Hash	½ cup	130
Strawberry	½ cup	110
Sundae, any flavor	4 oz.	160
ICE TEASERS (Nestlé)	8 fl. oz.	6

Food and Description	Measure or Quantity	Calories

J

JACK IN THE BOX
RESTAURANT:

Food and Description	Measure or Quantity	Calories
Beef fajita pita sandwich	6.2-oz. serving	333
Breadstick, sesame	.6-oz. piece	70
Breakfast Jack	4.4-oz. serving	307
Burger:		
Regular	3.6-oz. serving	267
Cheeseburger:		
Regular	4-oz. serving	315
Bacon	8.1-oz. serving	705
Double	5¼-oz. serving	467
Ultimate	9.9-oz. serving	942
Jumbo Jack:		
Regular	7.8-oz. serving	584
With cheese	8.5-oz. serving	677
Swiss & bacon	6.6-oz. serving	678
Cheesecake	3.5-oz. serving	309
Chicken fajita pita sandwich	6.7-oz. sandwich	292
Chicken fillet sandwich, grilled	7.2-oz. sandwich	408
Chicken strips	1 piece	87
Chicken supreme sandwich	8.1-oz. serving	575
Coffee, black	8 fl. oz.	2
Egg, scrambled, platter	8.8-oz. serving	662
Egg roll	1 piece	135
Fish supreme sandwich	8-oz. sandwich	554
French fries:		
Regular	2.4-oz. order	221
Large	3.8-oz. order	353
Jumbo	4.8-oz. order	442
Jelly, grape	.5-oz. serving	38
Ketchup	1 serving	10
Mayonnaise	1 serving	152
Milk, low fat	8 fl. oz.	122
Milk shake, any flavor	10 oz.	320
Mustard	1 serving	8
Onion rings	3.8-oz. serving	382
Orange juice	6.5-oz. serving	80
Pancake platter	8.1-oz. serving	612

Food and Description	Measure or Quantity	Calories
Salad:		
Chef	13-oz. salad	295
Mexican chicken	15.2-oz. salad	443
Side	3.9-oz. salad	51
Taco	14.8-oz. salad	641
Salad dressing:		
Regular:		
Blue cheese	1.2-oz. serving	131
Buttermilk	1.2-oz. serving	181
1000 Island	1.2-oz. serving	156
Dietetic or low calorie, French	1.2-oz. serving	80
Sauce:		
A-1	1.8-oz. serving	35
BBQ	.9-oz. serving	44
Guacamole	.9-oz. serving	55
Mayo-mustard	.8-oz. serving	124
Mayo-onion	.8-oz. serving	143
Salsa	.9-oz. serving	8
Seafood cocktail	1-oz. serving	32
Sweet & sour	1-oz. serving	40
Sausage crescent	5.5-oz. serving	585
Shrimp	1 piece (.3 oz.)	27
Soft drink:		
Sweetened:		
Coca-Cola Classic	12 fl. oz.	144
Dr Pepper	12 fl. oz.	144
Root beer, *Ramblin'*	12 fl. oz.	176
Sprite	12 fl. oz.	144
Diet *Coke*	12 fl. oz.	Tr.
Supreme crescent	5.1-oz. serving	547
Syrup, pancake	1.5-oz. serving	121
Taco:		
Regular	2.9-oz. serving	191
Super	4.8-oz. serving	288
Taquito	1-oz. piece	73
Tea, iced, plain	12 fl. oz.	3
Tortilla chips	1 oz.	139
Turnover, hot apple	4.2-oz. piece	410
JELL-O FRUIT BAR	1 bar	45
JELL-O FRUIT & CREAM BAR	1 bar	72
JELL-O GELATIN POPS	1 pop	35
JELL-O PUDDING POPS:		
Chocolate, chocolate with chocolate chips & vanilla with chocolate chips	1 bar	80
Chocolate covered chocolate & vanilla	1 bar	130

Food and Description	Measure or Quantity	Calories
JELLY, sweetened (See also individual flavors)		
(Crosse & Blackwell) all flavors	1 T.	51
JERUSALEM ARTICHOKE, pared	4 oz.	75
JOHANNISBERG RIESLING WINE (Louis M. Martini)	3 fl. oz.	59
JUST RIGHT, cereal (Kellogg's):		
With fiber nuggets	⅔ cup (1 oz.)	100
With fruit & nuts	¾ cup (1.3 oz.)	140

Food and Description	Measure or Quantity	Calories

K

Food and Description	Measure or Quantity	Calories
KABOOM, cereal (General Mills)	1 cup	110
KALE:		
Boiled, leaves only	4 oz.	110
Canned (Allen's) chopped, solids & liq.	½ cup	25
Frozen:		
(Bel-Air) cut	3.3 oz.	25
(Birds Eye) chopped	⅓ pkg.	32
(Frosty Acres)	3.3 oz.	25
(Southland) chopped	⅕ of 16-oz. pkg.	25
KARO SYRUP (See SYRUP)		
KEFIR (Alta-Dena Dairy):		
Plain	1 cup	180
Flavored	1 cup	190
KENMAI, cereal:		
Plain	¾ cup	110
Almond & raisin	¾ cup	150
KFC (KENTUCKY FRIED CHICKEN):		
Biscuit, buttermilk	2.3-oz. serving	235
Chicken:		
Original recipe:		
Breast:		
Center	3.6-oz. piece	260
Side	3.2-oz. piece	245
Drumstick	2-oz. piece	146
Thigh	3.7-oz. piece	294
Wing	1.9-oz. piece	178
Extra Tasty Crispy:		
Breast:		
Center	4.8 piece	344
Side	1 piece	379
Drumstick	2.4-oz. piece	205
Thigh	4.2-oz. piece	414
Wing	2.3-oz. piece	254
Hot & spicy:		
Breast:		
Center	4.3-oz. piece	382
Side	4.1-oz. piece	398

Food and Description	Measure or Quantity	Calories
Drumstick	2.5-oz. piece	207
Thigh	4.2-oz. piece	412
Wing	2.2-oz. piece	244
Skinfree crispy:		
Breast:		
Center	3.6-oz piece	244
Side	3.4-oz. piece	278
Drumstick	2.2-oz. piece	154
Thigh	2.9-oz. piece	235
Chicken Littles	1.7-oz. sandwich	169
Chicken nugget, *Kentucky Nuggets*	1 piece	46
Chicken sandwich, *Colonel's*	5.9-oz. sandwich	482
Cole slaw	3.2-oz. serving	114
Corn on the cob	2.5-oz. serving	90
Hot wings	.7-oz. piece	78
Potatoes:		
French fries	2.7-oz. regular order	244
Mashed, & gravy	3½-oz. serving	71
Sauce:		
Barbecue	1-oz. serving	35
Honey	.5-oz. serving	49
Mustard	1-oz. serving	36
Sweet & sour	1-oz. serving	58
KETCHUP (See CATSUP)		
KIDNEY:		
Beef, braised	4 oz.	286
Calf, raw	4 oz.	128
Lamb, raw	4 oz.	119
KIELBASA (See SAUSAGE, Polish-style)		
KING VITAMAN, cereal (Quaker)	1¼ cups (1 oz.)	113
KIPPER SNACKS (King David Brand) Norwegian	3¼-oz. can	195
KIWI FRUIT (Calavo)	1 fruit (5 oz., edible portion)	45
KIX, cereal	1½ cups (1 oz.)	110
KNOCKWURST (Hebrew National)	3 oz.	263
KOO KOOS (Dolly Madison)	1.5-oz. piece	190
KOOL-AID (General Foods):		
Canned, *Kool-Aid Koolers:*		
Cherry or mountainberry punch	8.45-fl.-oz. container	142
Grape	8.45-fl.-oz. container	136
Orange	8.45-fl.-oz. container	115

Food and Description	Measure or Quantity	Calories
Strawberry	8.45-fl.-oz. container	135
Tropical punch	8.45-fl.-oz. container	132
*Mix:		
Unsweetened, sugar to be added	8 fl. oz.	98
Pre-sweetened:		
Regular, sugar sweetened:		
Grape	8 fl. oz.	80
Orange, surfin' berry punch	8 fl. oz.	79
Purplesaurus rex, rainbow punch or tropical punch	8 fl. oz.	84
Dietetic, sugar free:		
Berry blue, cherry, grape or tropical punch	8 fl. oz.	3
Rainbow punch	8 fl. oz.	4
Raspberry	8 fl. oz.	2
KRISPIES, cereal (Kellogg's):		
Plain	1 cup	110
Frosted	¾ cup	110
Fruity marshmallow	1¼ cups	140
KUMQUAT, flesh & skin	5 oz.	74

Food and Description	Measure or Quantity	Calories

L

LAMB:
Leg:
Roasted, lean & fat	3 oz.	237
Roasted, lean only	3 oz.	158

Loin, one 5-oz. chop (weighed with bone before cooking) will give you:
Lean & fat	2.8 oz.	280
Lean only	2.3 oz.	122

Rib, one 5-oz. chop (weighed with bone before cooking) will give you:
Lean & fat	2.9 oz.	334
Lean only	2 oz.	118

Shoulder:
Roasted, lean & fat	3 oz.	287
Roasted, lean only	3 oz.	174

LASAGNA:
Dry:
(Buitoni) precooked	1 sheet	48
(Mueller's)	1 oz.	105

Canned:
(Chef Boyardee) microwave	7½-oz. serving	230
(Hormel) *Top Shelf*, Italian style	1 serving	360
(Nally's)	7½-oz. serving	180

Dietetic (Healthy Choice) with meat sauce | 7½-oz. serving | 220 |

Frozen:
(Banquet) *Family Entrees,* with meat sauce	¼ of 28-oz. pkg.	270
(Budget Gourmet) with meat sauce	9.4-oz. entree	300

(Buitoni):
Regular	9-oz. serving	342
Al forno	8-oz. serving	327
Meat sauce	5-oz. serving	212

(Celentano):
Regular	½ of 16-oz. pkg.	370

Food and Description	Measure or Quantity	Calories
Primavera	11-oz. pkg.	330
(Healthy Choice) with meat sauce	9-oz. meal	260
(Le Menu) healthy style entree,		
garden vegetable	10½-oz. entree	260
(Stouffer's):		
Regular, plain	10½-oz. meal	360
Lean Cuisine:		
With meat sauce	10¼-oz. meal	270
Zucchini	11-oz. meal	260
(Swanson):		
Homestyle Recipe, with meat		
sauce	10½-oz. entree	400
Hungry Man, with meat	18¾-oz. dinner	730
Main Course, with meat	13¼-oz. entree	450
(Ultra Slim Fast) vegetable	12-oz. meal	240
(Weight Watcher's):		
Garden	11-oz. meal	330
Italian cheese	11-oz. meal	380
LATKES, frozen (Empire Kosher):		
Mini	3-oz. serving	190
Triangles	3-oz. serving	140
LEEKS	4 oz.	59
LEMON:		
Whole	2⅛" lemon	22
Peeled	2⅛" lemon	20
LEMONADE:		
Canned:		
(Ardmore Farms)	6 fl. oz.	89
(Hi-C)	8.45-fl. oz. container	109
(Johanna Farms) *Ssips*	8.45-fl.-oz. container	85
Kool-Aid Koolers (General Foods)	8.45 fl.-oz. container	120
Chilled (Minute Maid) regular or pink	6 fl. oz.	81
*Frozen:		
Country Time, regular or pink	6 fl. oz.	62
(Sunkist)	6 fl. oz.	92
*Mix:		
Regular:		
Country Time, regular or pink	6 fl. oz.	62
(4C)	6 fl. oz.	60
(Funny Face)	6 fl. oz.	66
Kool-Aid, sweetened, regular or pink	6 fl. oz.	65

Food and Description	Measure or Quantity	Calories
(Pathmark) *No Frills*	8 fl. oz.	90
(Wyler's) regular	6 fl. oz.	61
Dietetic:		
Crystal Light	8 fl. oz.	5
Kool-Aid	6 fl. oz.	4
(Sunkist)	8 fl. oz.	8
LEMONADE BAR (Sunkist)	3-fl.-oz. bar	68
LEMON EXTRACT (Virginia Dare)	1 tsp.	21
LEMON JUICE:		
Canned, *ReaLemon*	1 fl. oz.	6
*Frozen (Sunkist) unsweetened	1 fl. oz.	7
LEMON-LIMEADE DRINK,		
Crystal Light	8 fl. oz.	4
LEMON PEEL, candied	1 oz.	90
LEMON & PEPPER SEASONING		
(Lawry's)	1 tsp.	6
LENTIL, cooked, drained	½ cup	107
LENTIL DINNER, canned (Health Valley) Fast Menu, with garden vegetables	7½ oz.	160
LETTUCE:		
Bibb or Boston	4" head	23
Cos or Romaine, shredded or broken into pieces	½ cup	4
Grand Rapids, Salad Bowl or Simpson	2 large leaves	9
Iceberg, New York or Great Lakes	¼ of 4¾" head	15
LIME, peeled	2" dia.	15
LIMEADE, frozen (Minute Maid)	6 fl. oz.	71
LIME JUICE, *ReaLime*	1 T.	2
LINGUINI, frozen:		
(Budget Gourmet):		
Regular, with shrimp	10-oz. meal	330
Slim Selects, with scallops & clams	9½-oz. meal	280
(Healthy Choice) with shrimp	9½-oz. meal	230
(Stouffer's) *Lean Cuisine*	9⅝-oz. meal	270
(Weight Watchers) seafood	9-oz. meal	210
***LITTLE CAESAR'S* RESTAURANT:**		
Crazy Bread	1 piece	98
Crazy Sauce	1 serving	63
Pizza:		
Baby Pan! Pan!	1 pizza	525
Round:		
Cheese:		
Small	1 slice	138
Medium	1 slice	154
Large	1 slice	169

Food and Description	Measure or Quantity	Calories
Cheese & pepperoni:		
Small	1 slice	151
Medium	1 slice	168
Large	1 slice	185
Slice! Slice!	1 slice	756
Square:		
Cheese, small	1 slice	188
Cheese & pepperoni, small	1 slice	204
Pizza meal, *Little Caesar's Meal:*		
Cheese & salad	1 serving	600
Green pepper, onion & mushroom, & salad	1 serving	640
Salad:		
Antipasto	12-oz. serving	170
Greek, small	1 serving	85
Sandwich:		
Ham & cheese	1 sandwich	520
Italian	1 sandwich	590
Tuna melt	1 sandwich	700
LIVER:		
Beef:		
Fried	6½" × 2⅜" × ⅜" slice	195
Cooked (Swift)	3.2-oz. serving	141
Calf, fried	6½" × 2⅛" × ⅜" slice	222
Chicken, simmered	2" × 2" × ⅝" piece	41
LIVERWURST SPREAD (Hormel)	1-oz. serving	70
LOBSTER:		
Canned, meat only	4-oz. serving	108
Cooked, meat only	1 cup	138
Frozen, South African lobster tail		
3 in 8-oz. pkg.	1 piece	87
4 in 8-oz. pkg.	1 piece	65
5 in 8-oz. pkg.	1 piece	51
LOBSTER NEWBURG, home recipe	1 cup	485
LOBSTER PASTE, canned, (USDA)	1-oz. serving	51
LOBSTER SALAD	4-oz. serving	125
LONG ISLAND TEA COCKTAIL (Mr. Boston) 12½% alcohol	3 fl. oz.	93
LONG JOHN SILVER'S RESTAURANT:		
Catfish:		
Dinner	13.2-oz. serving	860
Fillet	2½-oz. piece	180

Food and Description	Measure or Quantity	Calories
Catsup	.4-oz. packet	15
Chicken plank:		
Dinner:		
3-piece	13-oz. serving	830
4-piece	14.6-oz. serving	940
Single piece	1.6-oz. piece	110
Children's meals:		
Chicken planks	7.1-oz. serving	510
Fish	6½-oz. serving	440
Fish & chicken planks	8.1-oz. serving	550
Chowder, clam, with cod	7-oz. serving	140
Clam:		
Breaded	2.3-oz. serving	240
Dinner	12.8-oz. serving	980
Cod, entree, broiled	5.4-oz. serving	160
Cole slaw, drained on fork	3.4-oz. serving	140
Corn on the cob, with whirl	6.6-oz. ear	270
Cracker, *Club*	.2-oz. package	35
Fish, battered	2.6-oz. piece	150
Fish & chicken entree	14-oz. serving	870
Fish dinner, 3-piece	16.1-oz. serving	960
Fish dinner, home-style:		
3-piece	13.1-oz. serving	880
4-piece	14.8-oz. serving	1,010
6-piece	18.1-oz. serving	1,260
Fish & fries, entree:		
2-piece	10-oz. serving	660
3-piece	12.6-oz. serving	810
Fish, homestyle	1.6-oz. piece	125
Fish & more	13.4-oz. entree	800
Fish sandwich, homestyle	6.9-oz. serving	510
Fish sandwich platter, homestyle	13.4-oz. serving	870
Flounder, broiled	5.1-oz. piece	180
Gumbo, with cod & shrimp bobs	7-oz. serving	120
Halibut steak, broiled	4.1-oz. serving	140
Hushpuppie	.8-oz. piece	70
Pie:		
Lemon meringue	4.2-oz. slice	260
Pecan	4.4-oz. slice	530
Potato:		
Baked, without topping	7.1-oz. serving	150
Fries	3-oz. serving	220
Rice pilaf	3-oz. serving	150
Roll, dinner, plain	.9-oz. piece	70
Salad:		
Garden	8.7-oz. serving	170
Ocean chef	11.3-oz. serving	250

Food and Description	Measure or Quantity	Calories
Seafood, entree	11.9-oz. serving	270
Side	4.3-oz. serving	20
Salad dressing:		
Regular:		
Bleu cheese	1.5-oz packet	120
Ranch	1.5-oz. packet	140
Sea salad	1.6-oz. packet	140
Dietetic, Italian	1.6-oz. packet	18
Salmon, broiled	4.4-oz. piece	180
Sauce:		
Honey mustard	1.2-oz. packet	60
Seafood	1.2-oz. packet	45
Sweet & sour	1.2-oz. packet	60
Tartar	1-oz. packet	80
Seafood platter	14.1-oz. entree	970
Shrimp, battered	.5-oz. piece	40
Shrimp, breaded	2.2-oz. serving	190
Shrimp dinner, battered:		
6-piece	11.1-oz. serving	740
9-piece	12.6-oz. serving	860
Shrimp feast, breaded:		
13-piece	12.6-oz. serving	880
21-piece	14.8-oz. serving	1070
Shrimp, fish & chicken dinner	13.4-oz. dinner	840
Shrimp & fish dinner	12.3-oz. dinner	770
Shrimp scampi, baked entree	5.7-oz. meal	160
Vegetables, mixed	4-oz. serving	60
Vinegar, malt	.4-oz. packet	2
LOQUAT, fresh, flesh only	2 oz.	27
LUCKY CHARMS, cereal (General Mills)	1 cup (1 oz.)	110
LUNCHEON MEAT (See also individual listings such as BOLOGNA; HAM; etc.):		
Banquet loaf (Eckrich)	¾-oz. slice	50
Bar-B-Que loaf (Oscar Mayer)	1-oz. slice	46
Beef, jellied loaf (Hormel)	1.2-oz. slice	45
Gourmet loaf (Eckrich)	1-oz. slice	35
Ham & cheese (See HAM & CHEESE)		
Honey loaf:		
(Eckrich)	1-oz. slice	40
(Hormel)	1 slice	55
(Oscar Mayer)	1-oz. slice	34
Iowa Brand (Hormel)	1 slice	45
Jalapeño loaf (Oscar Mayer)	1-oz. slice	72
Liver cheese (Oscar Mayer)	1.3-oz. slice	114

Food and Description	Measure or Quantity	Calories
Liver loaf (Hormel)	1 slice	80
Luncheon loaf (Ohse)	1 oz.	75
Macaroni-cheese loaf (Eckrich)	1-oz. slice	68
Meat loaf	1-oz. serving	57
New England Brand sliced sausage:		
(Eckrich)	1-oz. slice	35
(Oscar Mayer) 92% fat free	.8-oz. slice	29
Old fashioned loaf (Oscar Mayer)	1-oz. slice	62
Olive loaf:		
(Eckrich)	1-oz. slice	80
(Hormel)	1-oz. slice	55
(Oscar Mayer)	1-oz. slice	60
Peppered loaf:		
(Eckrich)	1-oz. slice	40
(Hormel) *Light & Lean*	1 slice	50
(Oscar Mayer) 93% fat free	1-oz. slice	39
Pickle loaf:		
(Eckrich)	1-oz. slice	80
(Hormel)	1 slice	60
(Ohse)	1 oz.	60
Pickle & pimiento (Oscar Mayer)	1-oz. slice	62
Spiced (Hormel)	1 slice	75

Food and Description	Measure or Quantity	Calories

M

Food and Description	Measure or Quantity	Calories
MACADAMIA NUT		
(Royal Hawaiian)	1 oz.	197
MACARONI:		
Dry:		
Spinach (Creamette) ribbons	1 oz.	105
Whole wheat (Pritikin)	1 oz.	110
Cooked:		
8–10 minutes, firm	1 cup	192
14-20 minutes, tender	1 cup	155
Frozen:		
(Stouffer's)	5¾-oz. serving	170
(Swanson)	12-oz. dinner	370
MACARONI & CHEESE:		
Canned:		
(Franco-American)	7⅜-oz. serving	170
(Heinz)	7½-oz. serving	190
(Hormel) *Micro-Cup*	7½-oz. serving	189
(Ultra Slim Fast) microwaveable, zesty	8-oz. serving	230
Frozen:		
(Banquet):		
Casserole	8-oz. pkg.	350
Dinner	10-oz. dinner	420
(Birds Eye) For One	5¾-oz. pkg.	304
(Celentano) baked	½ of 12-oz. pkg.	290
(Green Giant) One Serving	5½-oz. entree	230
(Healthy Choice)	½ of 17-oz. pkg.	260
(Kraft)	12-oz. meal	610
(Stouffer's)	6-oz. serving	250
(Swanson)	12¼-oz. dinner	370
Mix:		
*(Kraft):		
Regular, plain	¼ box	190
Velveeta, shells	¼ box	270
*(Prince)	¾ cup	268
*(Town House)	1 cup	370
MACARONI & CHEESE LOAF, packaged (Ohse)	1 oz.	60
MACARONI & CHEESE PIE, frozen (Swanson)	7-oz. pie	200

Food and Description	Measure or Quantity	Calories
*MACARONI SALAD MIX (Betty Crocker) creamy	⅙ of pkg.	200
MACKEREL, Atlantic, broiled with fat	8½" × 2½" × ½" fillet	248
MAGIC SHELL (Smucker's)	1 T.	95
MAHI MAHI, frozen (Captain's Choice) fillet	3 oz.	73
MAI TAI COCKTAIL MIX (Holland House):		
Instant	.56-oz. envelope	64
Liquid	1 oz.	32
MALTED MILK MIX (Carnation):		
Chocolate	3 heaping tsps.	85
Natural	3 heaping tsps.	88
MALT LIQUOR:		
Colt 45	12 fl. oz.	156
Elephant	12 fl. oz.	212
Kingsbury (non-alcoholic)	12 fl. oz.	60
Mickey's	12 fl. oz.	156
Moussy (non-alcoholic)	12 fl. oz.	50
Schlitz	12 fl. oz.	176
MALT-O-MEAL, cereal	1 T.	33
MANDARIN ORANGE (See TANGERINE)		
MANGO, fresh	1 med. mango	88
MANGO NECTAR (Libby's)	6 fl. oz.	60
MANHATTAN COCKTAIL (Mr. Boston) 20% alcohol	3 fl. oz.	123
MANHATTAN COCKTAIL MIX (Holland House) liquid	1 oz.	28
MANICOTTI, frozen:		
(Budget Gourmet) with meat sauce	10-oz. meal	450
(Buitoni):		
Cheese	5.5 oz.	310
Florentine	2 manicotti	284
(Celentano):		
Without sauce	1 manicotti	85
With sauce	1 manicotti	150
(Le Menu) with three cheeses	11¾-oz. dinner	390
(Weight Watchers) cheese, in tomato sauce	9¼-oz. serving	300
*MANWICH (Hunt's):		
Regular	1 serving	320
Extra thick & chunky	1 serving	330
Mexican	1 serving	310
MAPLE SYRUP (See SYRUP, Maple)		

Food and Description	Measure or Quantity	Calories
MARGARINE:		
Regular:		
Heart Beat (GFA)	1 T.	25
I Can't Believe It's Not Butter	1 T.	90
(Imperial)	1 T.	100
(Land O' Lakes)	1 T.	100
(Mazola)	1 T.	100
(Parkay) regular, soft or		
squeeze	1 T.	101
(Shedd's)	1 T.	70
Imitation or dietetic:		
(Land O' Lakes):		
Soy oil spread	1 T.	75
With sweet cream:		
Stick	1 T.	90
Tub	1 T.	75
(Parkay)	1 T.	55
(Promise):		
Light, soft or stick	1 T.	70
Extra light, soft	1 T.	50
(Weight Watchers):		
Regular, reduced calorie	1 T.	60
Corn oil spread	1 T.	50
Light spread	1 T.	50
Sweet	1 T.	50
Whipped		
(Blue Bonnet; Miracle; Parkay)	1 T.	67
MARGARITA COCKTAIL:		
Canned (Mr. Boston) 12½%		
alcohol:		
Regular	3 fl. oz.	105
Strawberry	3 fl. oz.	138
*Frozen (Bacardi)	4 fl. oz.	82
Mix (Holland House):		
Dry:		
Regular	.5-oz. pkg.	57
Strawberry	.6-oz. pkg.	66
Liquid:		
Regular	1 fl. oz.	27
Strawberry	1 fl. oz.	31
MARINADE MIX:		
Chicken (Adolph's)	1-oz. packet	64
Meat:		
(French's)	1-oz. pkg.	80
(Kikkoman)	1-oz. pkg.	64
MARJORAM (French's)	1 tsp.	4

Food and Description	Measure or Quantity	Calories
MARMALADE:		
Sweetened:		
(Empress)	1 T.	52
(Home Brands)	1 T.	52
(Keiller)	1 T.	60
(Smucker's)	1 T.	54
Dietetic:		
(Estee; Louis Sherry)	1 T.	6
(Featherweight)	1 T.	16
(S&W) *Nutradiet*, red label	1 T.	12
MARSHMALLOW FLUFF	1 heaping tsp.	59
MARSHMALLOW KRISPIES,		
cereal (Kellogg's)	1¼ cups	140
MARTINI COCKTAIL (Mr. Boston):		
Gin, extra dry, 20% alcohol	3 fl. oz.	99
Vodka, 20% alcohol	3 fl. oz.	102
MASA HARINA (Quaker)	⅓ cup	137
MASA TRIGO (Quaker)	⅓ cup	149
MATZO (Manischewitz):		
Regular:		
Plain	1-oz piece	129
Egg	1 cracker	132
Miniature	1 cracker	9
Tam Tam	1 cracker	15
Dietetic:		
Tam Tam, unsalted	1 cracker	14
Thins	.8 oz. piece	91
MATZO FARFEL		
(Manischewitz)	½ cup	90
MAYONNAISE:		
Real:		
Blue Plate (Luzianne)	1 T.	100
Hellmann's (Best Foods)	1 T.	100
(Kraft)	1 T.	100
Imitation or dietetic:		
Blue Plate (Luzianne)	1 T.	50
(Estee)	1 T.	50
Heart Beat (GFA)	1 T.	40
Hellmann's (Best Foods)	1 T.	50
(Kraft) light	1 T.	45
(Pritikin) *Sweetlite*	1 T.	50
(Weight Watchers) any type	1 T.	50
MAYPO, cereal:		
30-second	¼ cup	89
Vermont style	¼ cup	121

Food and Description	Measure or Quantity	Calories
McDONALD'S:		
Big Mac	1 serving	560
Biscuit:		
With bacon, egg & cheese	1 order	440
With sausage	1 order	440
With sausage & egg	1 order	520
Cheeseburger	1 serving	310
Chicken McNuggets	1 serving	290
Chicken McNuggets Sauce:		
Barbecue	1.1-oz. serving	50
Honey	.5-oz. serving	45
Hot mustard	1.1-oz. serving	70
Cookies:		
Chocolate chip	1 package	330
McDonaldland	1 package	290
Danish:		
Apple or cheese, iced	1 piece	390
Cinnamon raisin	1 piece	440
Egg McMuffin	1 serving	290
Egg, scrambled	1 serving	140
English muffin, with butter	1 muffin	170
Filet-O-Fish	1 sandwich	440
Grapefruit juice	6 fl. oz.	80
Hamburger	1 serving	260
Hot cakes with butter & syrup	1 serving	410
McD.L.T.	1 sandwich	580
McLean Deluxe	7.3-oz. serving	320
Milk, 2% butterfat	8 fl. oz.	120
Orange juice	6 fl. oz.	80
Pie:		
Apple	1 pie	260
Cherry	1 pie	260
Potato:		
Fried	1 small order	220
Hash browns	1 order	130
Quarter Pounder:		
Regular	1 serving	410
With cheese	1 serving	520
Salad:		
Chef's	1 serving	230
Garden	1 serving	110
Side	1 serving	60
Salad bar:		
Bacon bits	1 packet	15
Chow mein noodles	1 packet	45
Croutons	1 packet	50

Food and Description	Measure or Quantity	Calories
Salad dressing:		
Blue cheese	1 packet (.5 oz.)	70
French	1 packet (.5 oz.)	58
1000 Island	1 packet (.5 oz.)	78
Lo-cal vinaigrette	1 packet (.5 oz.)	15
Sausage McMuffin:		
Plain	1 sandwich	370
With egg	1 sandwich	440
Sausage, pork	1 serving	180
Shake:		
Chocolate	1 serving	390
Strawberry	1 serving	350
Vanilla	1 serving	380
Soft drinks:		
Sweetened:		
Coca-Cola, Classic	12 fl. oz.	144
Orange drink	12 fl. oz.	133
Sprite	12 fl. oz.	144
Dietetic, *Diet Coke*	12 fl. oz.	1
Sundae:		
Caramel	1 serving	340
Hot fudge	1 serving	310
Strawberry	1 serving	280
Vanilla soft-serve, with cone	1 serving	140
*MEATBALL DINNER OR ENTREE, canned (Hunt's) *Minute Gourmet*	7.6-oz. serving	331
*MEATBALL SEASONING MIX (Durkee) Italian style	1 cup	619
MEATBALL STEW:		
Canned *Dinty Moore* (Hormel)	7½-oz. serving	245
Frozen (Stouffer's) *Lean Cuisine*	10-oz. serving	240
MEATBALLS, SWEDISH, frozen:		
(Armour) *Dinner Classics*	11¼-oz. meal	330
(Le Menu) healthy style	8-oz. entree	260
(Stouffer's) with noodles	11-oz. pkg.	480
MEAT LOAF DINNER, frozen:		
(Banquet):		
Cookin' Bags	4-oz. meal	200
Dinner	11-oz. dinner	440
(Budget Gourmet) Italian style	11-oz. meal	270
(Morton)	10-oz. dinner	310
(Swanson)	10¾-oz. dinner	360
(Ultra Slim Fast) & tomato sauce	10½-oz. meal	340
MEAT LOAF SEASONING MIX:		
*(Bell's)	4½ oz.	300
(Contadina)	3¾-oz. pkg.	360

Food and Description	Measure or Quantity	Calories
MEAT, POTTED:		
(Hormel)	1 T.	30
(Libby's)	1-oz. serving	55
MEAT TENDERIZER:		
Regular (Adolph's; McCormick)	1 tsp.	2
Seasoned (McCormick)	1 tsp.	5
MELBA TOAST, salted (Old London):		
Garlic, onion or white rounds	1 piece	10
Pumpernickel, rye, wheat or white	1 piece	17
MELON BALL, in syrup, frozen	½ cup	72
MENUDO, canned (Old El Paso)	½ can	476
MERLOT WINE (Louis M. Martini) 12½% alcohol	3 fl. oz.	63
MEXICALI DOGS, frozen (Hormel)	5-oz. serving	400
MEXICAN DINNER, frozen:		
(Patio) fiesta	12¼-oz. meal	470
(Swanson):		
Regular	14¼-oz. dinner	490
Hungry Man	20¼-oz. dinner	800
MILK, CONDENSED, *Eagle Brand* (Borden)	1 T.	64
***MILK, DRY,** non-fat, instant (Alba; Carnation; Pet; *Sanalac*)	1 cup	80
MILK, EVAPORATED:		
Regular:		
(Carnation)	1 fl. oz.	42
(Pet)	1 fl. oz.	43
Filled (Pet)	½ cup	150
Lowfat (Carnation)	1 fl. oz.	27
Skimmed (Carnation; *Pet 99*)	1 fl. oz.	25
MILK, FRESH:		
Buttermilk:		
(Friendship)	8 fl. oz.	120
(Lucerne):		
Regular	8 fl. oz.	120
Bulgarian	8 fl. oz.	150
Chocolate:		
(Borden) *Dutch Brand*	8 fl. oz.	180
(Hershey's) lowfat	8 fl. oz.	190
(Johanna Farms):		
Regular	8 fl. oz.	200
Lowfat	8 fl. oz.	150
(Land O' Lakes) lowfat:		
Regular	8 fl. oz.	150
With *Nutrasweet*	8 fl. oz.	110
(Lucerne) lowfat	8 fl. oz.	180

Food and Description	Measure or Quantity	Calories
(Nestlé) *Quik*	8 fl. oz.	220
Extra rich (Lucerne)	8 fl. oz.	170
Lowfat:		
(Borden):		
1% milkfat	8 fl. oz.	100
2% milkfat, *Hi-Protein Brand*	8 fl. oz.	140
(Johanna Farms):		
Regular:		
1% lowfat	8 fl. oz.	100
2% lowfat	8 fl. oz.	120
Buttermilk	8 fl. oz.	120
(Land O' Lakes):		
1% lowfat	8 fl. oz.	100
2% lowfat	8 fl. oz.	120
(Lucerne):		
Acidophilus:		
½, 1 or1½%	8 fl. oz.	90
2-10	8 fl. oz.	140
Skim:		
(Borden)	8 fl. oz.	90
(Land O' Lakes)	8 fl. oz.	90
Whole:		
(Borden) regular or high calcium	8 fl. oz.	150
(Johanna Farms)	8 fl. oz.	150
(Land O' Lakes)	8 fl. oz.	150
(Lucerne)	8 fl. oz.	150
MILK, GOAT, whole	1 cup	163
MILK, HUMAN	1 cup	163
MILK MAKERS (Swiss Miss):		
Chocolate, malted or strawberry	1 envelope or 1 tsp.	18
*Chocolate, malted or strawberry	8 fl. oz.	100
MILNOT, dairy vegetable blend	1 fl. oz.	38
MINERAL WATER (La Croix)	Any quantity	0
MINI-WHEATS, cereal (Kellogg's) frosted	1 biscuit	25
MINT LEAVES	½ oz.	4
MOLASSES:		
Barbados	1 T.	51
Blackstrap	1 T.	40
Dark (Brer Rabbit)	1 T.	33
Light	1 T.	48
Medium	1 T.	44
Unsulphured (Grandma's)	1 T.	70
MORNING FUNNIES, cereal (Ralston Purina)	1 cup	110
MORTADELLA SAUSAGE	1 oz.	89
MOST, cereal (Kellogg's)	½ cup (1 oz.)	100

Food and Description	Measure or Quantity	Calories
MOUSSE:		
Frozen (Weight Watchers):		
Chocolate	½ of 5-oz. container	170
Praline pecan	½ of 5.4-oz. container	190
Raspberry	½ of 5-oz. container	150
*Mix:		
Regular (Knorr):		
Unflavored	½ cup	80
Chocolate:		
Dark or milk	½ cup	90
White	½ cup	80
Dietetic:		
(Estee) any flavor	½ cup	70
Lite Whip (TKI Foods):		
Chocolate:		
With skim milk	½ cup	70
With whole milk	½ cup	80
Lemon or strawberry:		
With skim milk	½ cup	60
With whole milk	½ cup	70
(Weight Watchers)	½ cup	60
MÜESLIX, cereal (Kellogg's):		
Crispy blend	⅔ cup (1½ oz.)	160
Golden crunch	½ cup (1.2 oz.)	120
MUFFIN:		
Apple spice (Dunkin' Donuts)	1 piece	300
Blueberry:		
(Dunkin' Donuts)	3.6-oz. muffin	280
(Morton) rounds	1.5-oz. muffin	110
(Pepperidge Farm)	1 muffin	170
Bran (Pepperidge Farm)	1 muffin	170
Corn:		
(Dunkin' Donuts)	3.4-oz. muffin	340
(Morton)	1.7-oz. muffin	130
(Pepperidge Farm) frozen	1 muffin	180
Cranberry nut (Dunkin' Donuts)	3½-oz. muffin	290
English:		
Millbrook:		
Regular	2-oz. muffin	130
Whole wheat	2-oz. muffin	120
(Mrs. Wright's)	2-oz. muffin	130
(Pepperidge Farm):		
Plain	2-oz. muffin	140
Cinnamon, raisin	2-oz. muffin	150
(Pritikin) raisin	2.3-oz. muffin	150

Food and Description	Measure or Quantity	Calories
(Thomas'):		
Regular or frozen or sourdough	2-oz. muffin	133
Raisin	2.2-oz. muffin	153
(Wonder)	2-oz. muffin	130
Granola (Mrs. Wright's)	2.3-oz. muffin	150
Plain	1.4-oz. muffin	118
Raisin cinnamon (Mrs. Wright's)	2.3-oz. muffin	150
Sourdough (Wonder)	2-oz. muffin	130
MUFFIN MIX:		
*Apple cinnamon (Betty Crocker)	1/12 pkg.	120
*Applesauce, *Gold Medal* (General Mills)	1/6 pkg.	160
Blueberry:		
*(Betty Crocker) wild	1 muffin	120
(Duncan Hines) wild	1/12 pkg.	98
*Blueberry streusel (Betty Crocker)	1/12 pkg.	210
*Chocolate chip (Betty Crocker)	1/12 pkg.	150
*Cinnamon streusel (Betty Crocker)	1/10 pkg.	200
Cinnamon swirl (Duncan Hines) bakery style	1/12 pkg.	195
*Corn:		
(Dromedary)	1 muffin	120
Gold Medal (General Mills)	1/6 pkg.	130
Robin Hood (General Mills)	1/6 pkg.	130
Cranberry orange nut (Duncan Hines)	1/12 pkg.	184
*Honey bran, *Robin Hood* (General Mills)	1/6 pkg.	170
Oat bran:		
*(Betty Crocker)	1/8 pkg.	190
(Duncan Hines):		
Blueberry	1/12 pkg.	97
& honey	1/12 pkg.	129
*Oatmeal raisin (Betty Crocker)	1/12 pkg.	140
Pecan nut (Duncan Hines)	1/12 pkg.	211
MULLIGAN STEW, canned, *Dinty Moore, Short Orders* (Hormel)	7½-oz. can	230
MUSCATEL WINE (Italian Swiss Colony)	3 fl. oz.	93
MUSHROOM:		
Raw, whole	½ lb.	62
Raw, trimmed, sliced	½ cup	10
Canned (Green Giant) solids & liq., whole or sliced:		

Food and Description	Measure or Quantity	Calories
Regular	2-oz. serving	12
B&B	¼-oz. serving	12
Frozen:		
(Larsen)	3½ oz.	30
(Ore-Ida) breaded	2⅔ oz.	140
MUSHROOM, CHINESE, dried	1 oz.	81
MUSSEL, in shell	1 lb.	153
MUSTARD:		
Powder (French's)	1 tsp.	9
Prepared:		
Brown (French's; Gulden's)	1 tsp.	5
Chinese (Chun King)	1 tsp.	5
Dijon, *Grey Poupon*	1 tsp.	6
Horseradish (Nalley's)	1 tsp.	5
Yellow (Gulden's)	1 tsp.	5
MUSTARD GREENS:		
Canned (Allen's) solids & liq.	½ cup	20
Frozen:		
(Bel-Air)	3.3 oz.	20
(Birds Eye)	⅓ pkg.	25
(Frosty Acres)	3.3 oz.	20
MUSTARD SPINACH:		
Raw	1 lb.	100
Boiled, drained, no added salt	4-oz. serving	18

Food and Description	Measure or Quantity	Calories

N

NATHAN'S:
French fries	Regular order	550
Hamburger	1 sandwich	360
Hot dog & roll	1 order	290

NATURAL CEREAL:
Familia:
Regular	½ cup	187
Bran	½ cup	166
No added sugar	½ cup	181

Heartland:
Plain, coconut or raisin	¼ cup	130
Trail mix	¼ cup	120

Nature Valley (General Mills):
Cinnamon & raisin	⅓ cup	120
Fruit & nut or toasted oat	⅓ cup	130

NATURE SNACKS (Sun-Maid):
Carob Crunch	1 oz.	143
Carob Peanut	1¼ oz.	190
Carob Raisin or Yogurt Raisin	1¼ oz.	160
Tahitian Treat or Yogurt Crunch	1 oz.	123

NECTARINE, flesh only | 4 oz. | 73

NINTENDO CEREAL SYSTEM
(Ralston Purina)	1 cup	110

NOODLE:
Cooked, 1½" strips	1 cup	200
(Pennsylvania Dutch Brand) broad	1 oz. before cooking	105

NOODLE, CHOW MEIN:
(Chun King)	1 oz.	139
(La Choy)	½ cup (1 oz.)	150

NOODLE MIX:
*(Betty Crocker):
Fettucini Alfredo	¼ pkg.	220
Stroganoff	¼ pkg.	240

*(Lipton) & sauce:
Alfredo, carbonara	½ cup	131
Butter	½ cup	142
Cheese	½ cup	136
Chicken	½ cup	125

Food and Description	Measure or Quantity	Calories
Parmesan	½ cup	138
Stroganoff	½ cup	110
*NOODLE, RAMEN, canned (La Choy):		
Beef or oriental	1½ oz.	190
Chicken	1½ oz.	187
NOODLE, RICE (La Choy)	1 oz.	130
NOODLE ROMANOFF, frozen (Stouffer's)	⅓ pkg.	170
NOODLES & BEEF:		
Canned (Hormel) *Short Orders*	7½-oz. can	230
Frozen (Banquet) *Family Entree*	2-lb. pkg.	800
NOODLES & CHICKEN:		
Canned (Hormel) *Dinty Moore, Short Orders*	7½-oz. can	210
Frozen (Banquet)	10-oz. dinner	350
NUT (See specific type: CASHEW; MACADAMIA; etc.)		
NUT, MIXED:		
Dry roasted:		
(Flavor House)	1 oz.	172
(Party Pride)	1 oz.	170
(Planters) salted	1 oz.	160
Honey roasted (Fisher)	1 oz.	150
Oil roasted (Planters) with or without peanuts	1 oz.	180
NUT & HONEY CRUNCH, cereal (Kellogg's)	⅔ cup	110
NUTMEG (French's), ground	1 tsp.	11
NUTRAMENT, energy food, chocolate or vanilla	12 fl. oz.	360
NUTRIFIC, cereal (Kellogg's)	1 cup	120
NUTRI-GRAIN, cereal (Kellogg's):		
Almond raisin	⅔ cup	140
Raisin bran	1 cup	130
Wheat	⅔ cup	100

Food and Description	Measure or Quantity	Calories

O

OATBAKE, cereal (Kellogg's)	⅓ cup	110
OAT FLAKES, cereal (Post)	⅔ cup	107
OATMEAL:		
Cooked, regular	1 cup	132
Dry:		
Regular:		
(Elam's) Scotch style	1 oz.	108
(H-O) old fashioned	1 T.	14
(Safeway)	1 oz.	100
(3-Minute Brand)	⅓ cup	160
Instant:		
(H-O):		
Regular, boxed	1 T.	15
Apple cinnamon	1.2-oz. packet	130
Raisin & spice or sweet & mellow	1 packet	150
Oatmeal Swirlers (General Mills):		
Apple cinnamon, cinnamon spice or maple brown sugar	1 packet	160
Cherry or strawberry	1 packet	150
Milk chocolate	1 packet	170
(3-Minute Brand):	½-oz. packet	162
Plain	1-oz. packet	160
Apple & cinnamon	1⅜-oz. packet	210
Maple & brown sugar	1.5-oz. packet	220
Total (General Mills):		
Regular	1-oz. packet	110
Cinnamon raisin	1.8-oz. packet	140
Quick:		
(Ralston Purina)	⅓ cup	110
(Safeway)	1 oz.	100
(3-Minute Brand)	⅓ cup	110
Total (General Mills)	1 oz.	90
OATS & FIBER, cereal (H-O) hot:		
Boxed, dry	⅓ cup	100
Packets:		
Plain	1-oz. packet	110

Food and Description	Measure or Quantity	Calories
Raisin & bran	1.5-oz. packet	150
OIL, SALAD OR COOKING:		
(Bertoli) olive	1 T.	120
(Calavo) avocado	1 T.	120
(Country Pure) canola	1 T.	120
Crisco	1 T.	125
Heart Beat (GFA) canola oil	1 T.	180
Mazola, corn oil	1 T.	125
Mrs. Tucker's; (Goya)	1 T.	130
(Nu Made) salad or sunflower	1 T.	120
(Progresso) extra light, extra virgin or imported	1 T.	119
Sunlite, Wesson	1 T.	120
OKRA, frozen:		
(Bel-Air) whole	3.3 oz.	30
(Birds Eye) whole, baby	⅓ pkg.	36
(Frosty Acres):		
Cut	3.3 oz.	25
White	3.3 oz.	30
(Larsen) cut	3.3 oz.	25
(Ore-Ida) breaded	3 oz.	170
OLD FASHIONED COCKTAIL		
(Hiram Walker) 62 proof	3 fl. oz.	165
OLIVE:		
Green	4 med. or 3 extra large or 2 giant	19
Ripe (Lindsay) by size:		
Medium or small	.1-oz. olive	3
Extra large or large	.2-oz. olive	6
Colossal	.4-oz. olive	9
Super colossal	.5-oz. olive	11
OMELET, frozen (Swanson)		
TV Brand, Spanish style	7⅜-oz. entree	250
ONION:		
Raw	2½" onion	38
Boiled, pearl onion	½ cup	27
Canned (Durkee) *O & C:*		
Boiled	¼ of 16-oz. jar.	32
Creamed	¼ of 15½-oz. can	554
Dehydrated (Gilroy) flakes	1 tsp.	5
Frozen:		
(Birds Eye):		
Creamed	⅓ pkg.	106
Whole, small	⅓ pkg.	44
(Green Giant) in cheese sauce	½ cup	90
(Larsen):		
Diced	1 oz.	8

Food and Description	Measure or Quantity	Calories
Whole	3.3 oz.	35
(Mrs. Paul's) crispy rings	½ of 5-oz. pkg.	190
(Ore-Ida):		
Chopped	2 oz.	20
Dried-battered, *Onion Ringers*	2 oz.	140
ONION, COCKTAIL (Vlasic)	1 oz.	4
ONION, GREEN	1 small onion	4
ONION BOUILLON:		
(Herb-Ox)	1 cube	10
MBT	1 packet	16
(Wyler's) instant	1 tsp.	10
ONION SALAD SEASONING		
(French's) instant	1 T.	15
ONION SALT (French's)	1 tsp.	6
ONION SOUP (See SOUP, Onion)		
ORANGE, fresh:		
Peeled	½ cup	62
Sections	4 oz.	58
ORANGE DRINK:		
Canned:		
Bama (Borden)	8.45-fl.-oz. container	120
Capri Sun	6¾-fl.-oz. can	103
(Hi-C)	6 fl. oz.	95
(Lincoln)	6 fl. oz.	90
Ssips (Johanna Farms)	8.45-fl.-oz. container	130
*Mix:		
Regular (Funny Face)	8 fl. oz.	88
Dietetic:		
Crystal Light	6 fl. oz.	4
(Sunkist)	6 fl. oz.	6
ORANGE EXTRACT, imitation		
(Durkee)	1 tsp.	15
ORANGE FRUIT DRINK, canned		
(Ardmore Farms)	6 fl. oz.	86
ORANGE FRUIT JUICE BLEND,		
canned (Mott's)	9½-fl.-oz. can	139
ORANGE JUICE:		
Canned:		
(Borden) *Sippin' Pak*	8.45-fl.-oz. container	110
(Johanna Farms)	6 fl. oz.	84
(Land O' Lakes)	6 fl. oz.	90
(Minute Maid)	8.45-fl.-oz. container	129
(Ocean Spray)	6 fl. oz.	90

Food and Description	Measure or Quantity	Calories
(Town House)	6 fl. oz.	82
(Tree Top)	6 fl. oz.	90
Chilled (Sunkist)	6 fl. oz.	76
*Frozen:		
(Citrus Hill):		
Regular	6 fl. oz.	90
Lite	6 fl. oz.	60
(Minute Maid):		
Regular	6 fl. oz.	91
Calcium fortified	6 fl. oz.	93
Reduced acid	6 fl. oz.	89
(Sunkist)	6 fl. oz.	84
ORANGE JUICE BAR (Sunkist)	3-fl. oz. bar	72
ORANGE JUICE DRINK, canned, *Squeezit* (General Mills)	6⅜-oz. container	110
ORANGE PEEL, CANDIED	1 oz.	93
ORANGE-APRICOT JUICE COCKTAIL, *Musselman's*	8 fl. oz.	100
ORANGE-PINEAPPLE JUICE:		
Canned:		
(Land O' Lakes)	6 fl. oz.	90
(Texsun)	6 fl. oz.	90
ORANGE-PINEAPPLE-BANANA JUICE, canned (Land O' Lakes)	6 fl. oz.	100
ORCHARD BLEND JUICE, canned (Welch's):		
Apple-grape	6 fl. oz.	100
Harvest	6 fl. oz.	90
Vineyard	6 fl. oz.	120
OVALTINE, chocolate	¾ oz.	78
OVEN FRY (General Foods):		
Chicken:		
Extra crispy	4.2-oz. pkg.	461
Homestyle flour	3.2-oz. pkg.	339
Pork, *Shake & Bake,* extra crispy	4.2-oz. pkg.	482
OYSTER:		
Raw:		
Eastern	19-31 small or 13-19 med.	158
Pacific & Western	6-9 small or 4-6 med.	218
Canned (Bumble Bee) shelled, whole, solids & liq.	1 cup	218
Fried	4 oz.	271
OYSTER STEW, home recipe	½ cup	103

Food and Description	Measure or Quantity	Calories

P

PANCAKE, frozen:
  (Aunt Jemima):

Food and Description	Measure or Quantity	Calories
Original, microwave	1 pancake	70
Blueberry	1 pancake	73
Buttermilk, microwave:		
Regular	1 pancake	70
Lite	1 pancake	47
(Downyflake):		
Plain	1 pancake	93
Blueberry	1 pancake	96
(Pillsbury) microwave:		
Plain	1 pancake	83
Buttermilk	1 pancake	86
Wheat, harvest	1 pancake	80
(Weight Watchers)	2½-oz.-serving	140
*PANCAKE BATTER, frozen		
(Aunt Jemima):		
Plain	4" pancake	70
Blueberry or buttermilk	4" pancake	68
PANCAKE BREAKFAST, frozen:		
(Aunt Jemima):		
Homestyle, & sausages	6-oz. serving	420
Lite:		
With lite links, homestyle	6-oz. serving	310
With lite syrup	6-oz. serving	260
(Swanson) *Great Starts*:		
With bacon	4½-oz. serving	400
With sausage	6-oz. serving	460
Silver dollar, & sausage	3¾-oz. serving	310
(Weight Watchers):		
With blueberry topping	4¾-oz. serving	200
With links	4-oz. serving	220
With strawberry topping	4¾-oz. serving	200
*PANCAKE & WAFFLE MIX:		
Plain:		
(Aunt Jemima) Original	4" pancake	73
FastShake (Little Crow)	¼ of pkg.	133
Mrs. Butterworth's, butter flavor:		
Regular	4" pancake	73

Food and Description	Measure or Quantity	Calories
Complete (Pillsbury) *Hungry Jack:*	4" pancake	63
Complete, bulk	4" pancake	63
Extra Lights	4" pancake	70
Golden Blend, complete	4" pancake	80
Panshakes	4" pancake	83
Apple cinnamon, *Bisquick Shake 'N Pour* (General Mills)	4" pancake	90
Blueberry:		
Bisquick Shake 'N Pour (General Mills)	4" pancake	93
FastShake (Little Crow)	⅙ of 5-oz. container	84
(Pillsbury) *Hungry Jack*	4" pancake	107
Buttermilk:		
(Aunt Jemima) regular	4" pancake	100
(Betty Crocker) complete	4" pancake	70
Gold Medal (General Mills)	⅛ of mix	100
(Pillsbury) *Hungry Jack*, complete	4" pancake	63
Whole wheat (Aunt Jemima)	4" pancake	83
Dietetic:		
(Estee)	3" pancake	33
(Featherweight)	4" pancake	43
PANCAKE & WAFFLE SYRUP (See SYRUP, Pancake & Waffle)		
PAPAYA, fresh:		
Cubed	½ cup	36
Juice	4 oz.	78
PAPRIKA (French's)	1 tsp.	7
PARSLEY:		
Fresh, chopped	1 T.	2
Dried (French's)	1 tsp.	4
PASSION FRUIT, giant, whole	1 lb.	53
PASTA DINNER OR ENTREE:		
Canned (Franco-American):		
Circus O's, in tomato & cheese sauce	7⅜-oz. can	170
Sporty O's, with meatballs in tomato sauce	7⅜-oz. can	210
Teddy O's, in tomato & cheese sauce	7½-oz. can	170
Frozen:		
(Birds Eye):		
Continental	5-oz. serving	164
Primavera, For One	5-oz. serving	204

Food and Description	Measure or Quantity	Calories
(Budget Gourmet) Alfredo, with broccoli	5½-oz. serving	200
(Celentano) & cheese, baked	½ of 12-oz. pkg.	280
(Green Giant):		
Regular:		
Dijon	9½-oz. pkg.	260
Marinara, One Serving	6-oz. pkg.	180
Parmesan, with sweet peas, One Serving	5½-oz. pkg.	170
Pasta Accents:		
Creamy cheddar	⅙ of 16-oz. pkg.	100
Garlic	⅙ of 16-oz. pkg.	110
Primavera	⅙ of 16-oz. pkg.	110
(Healthy Choice):		
Primavera	11-oz. meal	280
With shrimp	12½-oz. meal	360
(Stouffer's):		
Carbonara	9¾-oz. meal	620
Mexicali	10-oz. meal	490
Primavera	10⅝-oz. meal	270
(Weight Watchers):		
Regular, angel hair	10-oz. meal	200
Smart Ones, portofino	9½-oz. meal	160
Ultimate 200, Italiano	8-oz. meal	160
PASTA SALAD:		
*Mix (Betty Crocker) *Suddenly Salads,* Italian	⅙ pkg.	160
*Mix *Salad Bar Pasta* (Buitoni):		
Country Buttermilk	⅙ pkg.	250
Italian Creamy	⅙ pkg.	290
Frozen (Birds Eye) classic, Italian style	½ of 10-oz. pkg.	170
***PASTA & SAUCE,** mix (Lipton):		
Cheese supreme	¼ pkg.	139
Mushroom & chicken	¼ pkg.	124
Oriental, with fusilli	¼ pkg.	130
Tomato, herb	¼ pkg.	130
PASTINAS, egg	1 oz.	109
PASTRAMI, packaged:		
(Carl Buddig) smoked, sliced	1 oz.	40
Hebrew National, first cut	1 oz.	44
PASTRY POCKETS (Pillsbury)	1 pocket	240
PASTRY SHEET, PUFF, frozen (Pepperidge Farm)	1 sheet	1040
PASTRY SHELL, frozen (Pet-Ritz)	3" tart shell	150
PÂTÉ:		
De foie gras	1 T.	69

Food and Description	Measure or Quantity	Calories
Liver:		
(Hormel)	1 T.	35
(Sell's)	1 T.	93
PDQ, milk flavoring:		
Chocolate	1 T.	66
Strawberry	1 T.	60
PEA, CROWDER, frozen		
(Southland)	⅕ of 16-oz. pkg.	130
PEA, GREEN:		
Boiled	½ cup	58
Canned, regular pack, solids & liq.:		
(Green Giant):		
Early with onions, sweet or		
sweet with onions	¼ of 17-oz. can	60
Sweet, mini	¼ of 17-oz. can	64
(Larsen) *Fresh-Lite*	½ cup	50
(Town House)	½ cup	70
Canned, dietetic pack, solids & liq.:		
(Del Monte) no salt added, sweet	½ cup	60
(Diet Delight)	½ cup	50
(Featherweight) sweet	½ cup	70
(Larsen) *Fresh-Lite*, low sodium	½ cup	50
(Pathmark)	½ cup	70
Frozen:		
(Bel-Air)	3.3 oz.	80
(Birds Eye):		
Regular	⅓ pkg.	78
In butter sauce	⅓ pkg.	85
In cream sauce	⅓ pkg.	84
(Frosty Acres):		
Regular	3.3 oz.	80
Tiny	3.3 oz.	60
(Green Giant):		
In cream sauce	½ cup	100
Sweet, *Harvest Fresh*	½ cup	80
(Le Sueur) in butter sauce	3.3 oz.	67
PEA & CARROT:		
Canned, regular pack, solids & liq.:		
(Comstock)	½ cup	60
(Del Monte)	½ cup	50
(Libby's)	½ cup	56
(Veg-All)	½ cup	50
Canned, dietetic pack, solids & liq.:		
(Diet Delight)	½ cup	40
(Larsen) *Fresh-Lite*, low sodium	½ cup	50
(S&W) *Nutradiet*	½ cup	35

Food and Description	Measure or Quantity	Calories
Frozen:		
(Bel-Air)	3.3 oz.	60
(Birds Eye)	⅓ pkg.	61
(McKenzie)	3.3-oz. serving	60
PEA POD:		
Boiled, drained solids	4 oz.	49
Frozen (La Choy)	6-oz. pkg.	70
PEACH:		
Fresh, with thin skin	2" dia.	38
Fresh slices	½ cup	32
Canned, regular pack, solids & liq.:		
(Country Pure)	½ cup	50
(Hunt's)	4-oz.	80
Canned, dietetic pack, solids & liq.:		
(Del Monte) Lite, Cling	½ cup	50
(Diet Delight) Cling:		
Juice pack	½ cup	50
Water Pack	½ cup	30
(Featherweight):		
Cling or Freestone, juice pack	½ cup	50
Cling, water pack	½ cup	30
(S&W) *Nutradiet,* Cling:		
Juice pack	½ cup	60
Water pack	½ cup	30
Dried (Town House)	2 oz.	140
Frozen (Birds Eye)	5-oz. pkg.	141
PEACH BUTTER (Smucker's)	1 T.	45
PEACH DRINK, canned (Hi-C)	6 fl. oz.	101
PEACH JUICE, canned (Smucker's)	8 fl. oz.	120
PEACH LIQUEUR (DeKuyper)	1 fl. oz.	82
PEACH NECTAR, canned		
(Ardmore Farms)	6 fl. oz.	90
PEACH PARFAIT, frozen		
(Pepperidge Farm)	4½ oz.	150
PEACH PRESERVE OR JAM:		
Sweetened:		
(Bama)	1 T.	45
(Home Brands)	1 T.	50
(Smucker's)	1 T.	54
Dietetic (Dia-Mel)	1 T.	6
PEANUT:		
In shell (Planters)	1 oz.	160
Roasted:		
(Beer Nuts)	1 oz.	180
(Eagle):		
Fancy Virginia	1 oz.	180
Honey roast	1 oz.	170

Food and Description	Measure or Quantity	Calories
Lightly salted	1 oz.	170
(Fisher):		
Dry, salted or unsalted	1 oz.	160
Honey	1 oz.	150
Oil:		
Blanched	1 oz.	160
Party	1 oz.	170
(Guy's) dry	1 oz.	170
(Planters):		
In shell	1 oz.	160
Shelled:		
Dry, salted	1 oz.	160
Honey	1 oz.	170
Oil:		
Regular or tavern	1 oz.	170
Sweet 'n Crunchy	1 oz.	140
(Weight Watchers)	1 pouch	100
PEANUT, SPANISH		
(Fisher):		
Raw	1 oz.	160
Roasted, oil	1 oz.	170
(Party Pride)	1 oz.	180
(Planters):		
Raw	1 oz.	150
Roasted:		
Dry	1 oz.	160
Oil	1 oz.	170
PEANUT BUTTER:		
Regular:		
(Algood) any type	1 T.	95
(Holsum)	1 T.	94
(Home Brands)	1 T.	105
Jif	1 T.	93
(Nu Made) chunky or creamy	1 T.	95
(Pathmark) regular or *No Frills*	1 T.	100
(Peter Pan)	1 T.	90
(Skippy) creamy or super chunk	1 T.	95
(Smucker's)	1 T.	100
Dietetic or low sodium:		
(Estee) low sodium	1 T.	100
(Health Valley) no salt, chunky	1 T.	90
(Home Brands):		
Lightly salted or unsalted	1 T.	105
No sugar added	1 T.	90
(Peter Pan) creamy	1 T.	95
(S&W) *Nutradiet,* low sodium	1 T.	93
(Smucker's) low sodium	1 T.	100

Food and Description	Measure or Quantity	Calories
PEANUT BUTTER BAKING CHIPS (Reese's)	3 T. (1 oz.)	153
PEANUT BUTTER & JELLY (Bama)	1 T.	75
PEAR:		
Fresh	3" × 2½" pear	101
Canned, regular pack, solids & liq.:		
(Country Pure)	½ cup	60
(Libby's)	½ cup	102
Canned, dietetic pack, solids & liq.:		
(Featherweight) Bartlett:		
Juice pack	½ cup	60
Water pack	½ cup	40
(Hunt's) halves	4 oz.	90
(Libby's) water pack	½ cup	60
(Pathmark) Bartlett, halves	½ cup	90
Dried (Sun-Maid)	½ cup	260
PEAR, STRAINED (Larsen)	½ cup	65
PEAR-APPLE JUICE (Tree Top)	6 fl. oz.	90
PEAR-GRAPE JUICE (Tree Top)	6 fl. oz.	100
PEAR NECTAR, canned (Ardmore Farms)	6 fl. oz.	96
PEAR-PASSION FRUIT NECTAR, canned (Libby's)	6 fl. oz.	100
PEBBLES, cereal (Post)	⅞ cup (1 oz.)	113
PECAN:		
Halves	6-7 pieces	48
Roasted, dry:		
(Fisher) salted	1 oz.	220
(Planters)	1 oz.	190
PECTIN, FRUIT:		
Certo	.6-oz. pkg.	19
Sure-Jell	1¾-oz. pkg.	170
PEPPER BLACK (French's):		
Regular	1 tsp.	9
Seasoned	1 tsp.	8
PEPPER, BANANA (Vlasic) hot rings	1 oz.	4
PEPPER, CHERRY (Vlasic) mild	1 oz.	8
PEPPER, CHILI, canned:		
(Del Monte):		
Green, whole	½ cup	20
Jalapeño or chili, whole	½ cup	30
(Old El Paso) green, chopped or whole	1 oz.	7
(Ortega):		
Diced, strips or whole	1 oz.	10

Food and Description	Measure or Quantity	Calories
Jalapeño, diced or whole	1 oz.	9
(Vlasic) Jalapeño	1 oz.	8
PEPPER, SWEET:		
Raw:		
Green:		
Whole	1 lb.	82
Without stem & seeds	1 med. pepper (2.6 oz.)	13
Red:		
Whole	1 lb.	112
Without stem & seeds	1 med. pepper (2.2 oz.)	19
Boiled, green, without salt, drained	1 med. pepper (2.6 oz.)	13
Frozen:		
(Frosty Acres) diced:		
Green	1 oz.	6
Red & green	1 oz.	7
(Larsen) green	1 oz.	6
(Southland) diced	2-oz. serving	10
PEPPER, STUFFED:		
Home recipe	2¾" × 2½" pepper with 1⅛ cups stuffing	314
Frozen:		
(Celentano)	12½-oz. pkg.	290
(Stouffer's) green	7¾-oz. serving	200
(Weight Watchers) with veal stuffing	11⅜-oz. meal	270
PEPPER & ONION, frozen (Southland)	2-oz. serving	15
PEPPER STEAK:		
*Canned (La Choy)	⅜ cup	210
Frozen:		
(Armour) *Classics Lite,* beef	11¼-oz. dinner	220
(Healthy Choice) beef:		
Dinner	11-oz. dinner	290
Entree	9½-oz. entree	250
(La Choy) *Fresh & Lite*, with rice & vegetables	10-oz. meal	280
(Le Menu)	11½-oz. dinner	370
(Stouffer's)	10½-oz. serving	330
PEPPERMINT EXTRACT, imitation (Durkee)	1 tsp.	15
PEPPERONCINI (Vlasic) Greek, mild	1 oz.	4

Food and Description	Measure or Quantity	Calories
PEPPERONI:		
(Eckrich)	1-oz. serving	135
(Hormel) regular or Rosa Grande	1-oz. serving	140
PERCH, OCEAN:		
Atlantic, raw:		
Whole	1 lb.	124
Meat only	4 oz.	108
Pacific, raw, whole	1 lb.	116
Frozen:		
(Captain's Choice) fillet	3 oz.	103
(Frionor) *Norway Gourmet*	4 oz. fillet	120
(Mrs. Paul's) fillet, breaded & fried	2-oz. piece	145
(Van de Kamp's) batter dipped, french fried	2-oz. piece	135
PERNOD (Julius Wile)	1 fl. oz.	79
PERSIMMON:		
Japanese or Kaki, fresh:		
With seeds	4.4-oz. piece	79
Seedless	4.4-oz. piece	81
Native, fresh, flesh only	4-oz. serving	144
PETITE SIRAH WINE (Louis M. Martini) 12% alcohol	3 fl. oz.	61
PHEASANT, raw, meat only	4-oz. serving	184
PICKLE:		
Cucumber, fresh or bread & butter:		
(Fannings)	1.2-oz. serving	17
(Featherweight) low sodium	1-oz. pickle	12
(Vlasic):		
Chips	1 oz.	7
Stix, sweet butter	1 oz.	5
Dill:		
(Featherweight) low sodium, whole	1-oz. serving	4
(Smucker's):		
Hamburger, sliced	1 slice	Tr.
Polish, whole	3½" pickle	8
(Vlasic):		
Original	1 oz.	2
No garlic	1 oz.	4
Hamburger (Vlasic) chips	1-oz. serving	2
Hot & spicy (Vlasic) garden mix	1 oz.	4
Kosher dill:		
(Claussen) halves or whole	2-oz. serving	7
(Featherweight) low sodium	1-oz. serving	4
(Smucker's):		
Baby	2⅜"-long pickle	4

Food and Description	Measure or Quantity	Calories
Whole	3½"-long pickle	8
(Vlasic)	1 oz.	4
Sweet:		
(Nalley's) *Nubbins*	1-oz. serving	28
(Smucker's):		
Gherkins	2"-long pickle	15
Whole	2½"-long pickle	18
(Vlasic)	1 oz.	30
Sweet & sour (Claussen) slices	1 slice	3
PIE:		
Regular, non-frozen:		
Apple:		
Home recipe, two-crust	⅙ of 9" pie	404
(Dolly Madison)	4½-oz. pie	490
(Entenmann's) homestyle	2.1 oz.	140
Banana, home recipe, cream or custard	⅙ of 9" pie	336
Blackberry, home recipe, two-crust	⅙ of 9" pie	384
Blueberry:		
Home recipe, two-crust	⅙ of 9" pie	382
(Dolly Madison)	4½-oz. pie	430
Boston cream, home recipe	1/12 of 8" pie	208
Butterscotch, home recipe, one-crust	⅙ of 9" pie	406
Cherry:		
Home recipe, two-crust	⅙ of 9" pie	412
(Dolly Madison) regular	4½-oz. pie	470
Chocolate (Dolly Madison):		
Regular	4½-oz. pie	560
Pudding	4½-oz. pie	500
Chocolate chiffon, home recipe	⅙ of 9" pie	459
Chocolate meringue, home recipe	⅙ of 9" pie	353
Coconut custard, home recipe	⅙ of 9" pie	357
Coconut custard (Entenmann's)	1.8 oz.	140
Lemon meringue, home recipe, one-crust	⅙ of 9" pie	357
Mince, home recipe, two-crust	⅙ of 9" pie	428
Peach (Dolly Madison)	4½-oz. pie	460
Pumpkin, home recipe, one-crust	⅙ of 9" pie	321
Raisin, home recipe, two-crust	⅙ of 9" pie	427
Vanilla (Dolly Madison) pudding	4½-oz. pie	500
Frozen:		
Apple:		
(Banquet) family size	⅙ of 20-oz. pie	250

Food and Description	Measure or Quantity	Calories
(Mrs. Smith's):		
Regular:		
Plain	⅛ of 8" pie	220
Dutch	⅛ of 10" pie	430
Natural Juice, dutch	⅛ of 9" pie	380
Pie in Minutes	⅛ of 25-oz. pie	210
(Pet-Ritz)	⅙ of 26-oz. pie	330
(Weight Watchers)	3½ oz.	200
Banana cream:		
(Banquet)	⅙ of 14-oz. pie	180
(Pet-Ritz)	⅙ of 14-oz. pie	170
Blackberry (Banquet)	⅙ of 20-oz. pie	270
Blueberry:		
(Banquet)	⅙ of 20-oz. pie	266
(Mrs. Smith's):		
Regular	⅛ of 26-oz. pie	210
Pie in Minutes	⅛ of 25-oz. pie	220
(Pet-Ritz)	⅙ of 26-oz. pie	370
Cherry:		
(Banquet)	⅙ of 20-oz. pie	250
(Mrs. Smith's):		
Regular	⅛ of 46-oz. pie	390
Natural Juice	⅛ of 36.8-oz pie	350
(Pet-Ritz)	⅙ of 26-oz. pie	300
Chocolate cream:		
(Banquet)	⅙ of 14-oz. pie	190
(Pet-Ritz)	⅙ of 14-oz. pie	190
Coconut cream (Banquet)	⅙ of 14-oz. pie	190
Coconut custard (Mrs. Smith's)	⅛ of 25-oz. pie	180
Custard, egg (Pet-Ritz)	⅙ of 24-oz. pie	200
Lemon cream:		
(Banquet)	⅙ of 14-oz. pie	168
(Pet-Ritz)	⅙ of 14-oz. pie	190
Mince:		
(Banquet)	⅙ of 20-oz. pie	260
(Mrs. Smith's)	⅛ of 46-oz. pie	430
(Pet-Ritz)	⅙ of 26-oz. pie	280
Mississippi mud (Pepperidge Farm)	2¼ oz.	310
Peach:		
(Banquet)	⅙ of 20-oz. pie	245
(Mrs. Smith's):		
Regular	⅛ of 46-oz. pie	360
Natural Juice	⅛ of 36.8-oz. pie	330
(Pet-Ritz)	⅙ of 26-oz. pie	320
Pumpkin:		
(Banquet)	⅙ of 20-oz. pie	200

Food and Description	Measure or Quantity	Calories
(Mrs. Smith's) *Pie In Minutes*	⅛ of 25-oz. pie	190
Strawberry cream (Banquet)	⅙ of 14-oz. pie	170
PIECRUST:		
Home recipe, 9" pie	1 crust	900
Frozen:		
(Empire Kosher)	7-oz. shell	1001
(Mrs. Smith's):		
8" shell	10 oz.	640
9" shell, shallow	10 oz.	640
9⅝" shell	15 oz.	960
(Oronoque):		
Regular	7.4 oz.	1020
Deep dish	8½ oz.	1200
(Pet-Ritz):		
Regular	⅙ of 5-oz. pkg.	110
Deep dish:		
Regular	⅙ of 6-oz. pkg.	130
All vegetable shortening	⅙ of 6-oz. pkg.	140
Graham cracker	⅙ of 5-oz. pkg.	110
Refrigerated (Pillsbury)	2 crusts	1920
*PIECRUST MIX:		
(Betty Crocker):		
Regular	1/16 pkg.	120
Stick	⅛ stick	120
(Flako)	⅙ of 9" pie shell	245
(Pillsbury) mix or stick	⅙ of 2-crust pie	270
PIE FILLING (See also PUDDING OR PIE FILLING):		
Apple:		
(Comstock)	⅙ of 21-oz. can	110
(Thank You Brand)	3½ oz.	91
(White House)	½ cup	163
Apple rings or slices (See APPLE, canned)		
Apricot (Comstock)	⅙ of 21-oz. can	110
Banana cream (Comstock)	⅙ of 21-oz. can	110
Blueberry (Comstock)	⅙ of 21-oz. can	120
Cherry (White House)	3½ oz.	99
Coconut cream (Comstock)	⅙ of 21-oz. can	120
Coconut custard, home recipe, made with egg yolk & milk	5 oz. (inc. crust)	288
Lemon (Comstock)	⅙ of 21-oz. can	160
Mincemeat (Comstock)	½ of 21-oz. can	170
Peach (White House)	½ cup	158
Pumpkin (Libby's) (See also PUMPKIN, canned)	1 cup	210
Raisin (Comstock)	⅙ of 21-oz. can	140

Food and Description	Measure or Quantity	Calories
*PIE MIX:		
Boston Cream (Betty Crocker)	⅛ of pie	270
Chocolate (Royal)	⅛ of pie	260
PIEROGIES, frozen:		
(Empire Kosher):		
Cheese	1½ oz.	110
Onion	1½ oz.	90
(Mrs. Paul's) potato & cheese	1 piece	90
PIGS FEET, pickled	4-oz. serving	226
PIMIENTO, canned:		
(Dromedary) drained	1-oz. serving	10
(Ortega)	¼ cup	6
(Sunshine) diced or sliced	1 T.	4
PIÑA COLADA (Mr. Boston)		
12½% alcohol	3 fl. oz.	249
PIÑA COLADA MIX:		
*(Bacardi) frozen	4 fl. oz.	110
*(Bar-Tender's)	5 fl. oz.	254
(Holland House):		
Dry mix	.56-oz. pkg.	82
Liquid mix	1 fl. oz.	33
PINEAPPLE:		
Fresh, chunks	½ cup	52
Canned, regular pack, solids & liq.:		
(Dole):		
Heavy syrup, chunk, crushed or sliced	½ cup	90
Juice pack, chunk, crushed or sliced	½ cup	70
(Town House) juice pack	½ cup	70
Canned, unsweetened or dietetic, solids & liq.:		
(Diet Delight) juice pack	½ cup	70
(Libby's) Lite	½ cup	60
(S&W) *Nutradiet*	1 slice	30
PINEAPPLE, CANDIED	1-oz. serving	90
PINEAPPLE FLAVORING, imitation		
(Durkee)	1 tsp.	6
PINEAPPLE & GRAPEFRUIT JUICE DRINK, canned:		
(Del Monte) regular or pink	6 fl. oz.	90
(Dole) pink	6 fl. oz.	101
(Texsun)	6 fl. oz.	91
*PINEAPPLE GRAPEFRUIT JUICE, frozen (Dole)	6 fl. oz.	90

Food and Description	Measure or Quantity	Calories
PINEAPPLE JUICE:		
Canned:		
(Dole)	6 fl. oz.	100
(Minute Maid) On the Go	10-fl.-oz. bottle	165
(Mott's)	9.5-fl.-oz. can	169
(Pathmark) regular or *No Frills*	6 fl. oz.	100
(Town House)	6 fl. oz.	100
(Tree Top)	6 fl. oz.	100
*Frozen (Minute Maid)	6 fl. oz.	99
PINEAPPLE-ORANGE JUICE:		
Canned:		
(Dole)	6 fl. oz.	100
(Johanna Farms) *Tree Ripe*	8.45-fl.-oz. container	132
*Frozen (Minute Maid)	6 fl. oz.	98
PINEAPPLE PRESERVE OR JAM, sweetened (Home Brands)	1 T.	52
PINE NUT, pignolias, shelled	1 oz.	156
PINOT CHARDONNAY WINE (Paul Masson) 12% alcohol	3 fl. oz.	71
PISTACHIO NUT:		
In shell	½ cup	197
Shelled	¼ cup	184
(Fisher) shelled, roasted, salted	1 oz.	174
PIZZA HUT:		
Hand-tossed, medium size:		
Cheese	1 slice	259
Pepperoni	1 slice	250
Super supreme	1 slice	231
Supreme	1 slice	270
Pan, medium size:		
Cheese	1 slice	246
Pepperoni	1 slice	270
Super supreme	1 slice	281
Supreme	1 slice	294
Personal Pan Pizza:		
Pepperoni	9-oz. pizza	675
Supreme	9.3-oz. pizza	647
Thin 'n Crispy, medium size:		
Cheese	1 slice	199
Pepperoni	1 slice	206
Super Supreme	1 slice	232
Supreme	1 slice	229
PIZZA PIE (See also *LITTLE CAESAR'S* or *SHAKEY'S*):		
Regular, non-frozen:		
Home recipe	⅛ of 14" pie	177

Food and Description	Measure or Quantity	Calories
(Domino's):		
Beef, ground:		
Plain:		
12" pizza (small)	1 slice	216
16" pizza (large)	1 slice	303
With pepperoni:		
12" pizza (small)	1 slice	216
16" pizza (large)	1 slice	303
Cheese:		
Plain:		
12" pizza (small)	1 slice	157
16" pizza (large)	1 slice	239
Double cheese:		
12" pizza (small)	1 slice	240
16" pizza (large)	1 slice	350
Double, with pepperoni		
12" pizza (small)	1 slice	227
16" pizza (large)	1 slice	389
Mushroom & sausage:		
12" pizza (small)	1 slice	183
16" pizza (large)	1 slice	266
Pepperoni:		
Plain:		
12" pizza (small)	1 slice	192
16" pizza (large)	1 slice	278
With mushrooms:		
12" pizza (small)	1 slice	194
16" pizza (large)	1 slice	280
With sausage:		
12" pizza (small)	1 slice	215
16" pizza (large)	1 slice	303
Sausage:		
12" pizza (small)	1 slice	180
16" pizza (large)	1 slice	264
(Godfather's):		
Cheese:		
Original:		
Mini	¼ of pizza (2.8 oz.)	190
Small	⅙ of pizza (3.6 oz.)	240
Medium	⅛ of pizza (4½ oz.)	270
Large:		
Regular	¹⁄₁₀ of pizza (4.4 oz.)	297
Hot slice	⅛ of pizza (5½ oz.)	370
Stuffed:		
Small	⅙ of pizza (4.4 oz.)	310
Medium	⅛ of pizza (4.8 oz.)	350
Large	¹⁄₁₀ of pizza (5.2 oz.)	381

Food and Description	Measure or Quantity	Calories
Thin crust:		
Small	⅙ of pizza (2.6 oz.)	180
Medium	⅛ of pizza (3 oz.)	210
Large	⅒ of pizza (3.4 oz.)	228
Combo:		
Original:		
Mini	¼ of pizza (3.8 oz.)	240
Small	⅙ of pizza (5.6 oz.)	360
Medium	⅛ of pizza (6.2 oz.)	400
Large:		
Regular	⅒ of pizza (6.8 oz.)	437
Hot slice	⅛ of pizza (8.5 oz.)	550
Stuffed:		
Small	⅙ of pizza (6.3 oz.)	430
Medium	⅛ of pizza (7 oz.)	480
Large	⅒ of pizza (7.6 oz.)	521
Thin crust:		
Small	⅙ of pizza (4.3 oz.)	270
Medium	⅛ of pizza (4.9 oz.)	310
Large	⅒ of pizza (5.4 oz.)	336
Frozen:		
Bacon (Totino's)	½ of 10-oz. pie	370
Bagel (Empire Kosher)	2-oz. serving	140
Canadian style bacon:		
(Jeno's) crisp 'n tasty	½ of 7.7-oz. pie	250
(Stouffer's) french bread	½ of 11⅝-oz. pkg.	360
(Totino's)	½ of 10.2-oz. pkg.	310
Cheese:		
(Celentano):		
Mini slice	1 slice	150
Thick crust	⅓ of 13-oz. pie	290
(Empire Kosher):		
Regular	⅓ of 10-oz. pie	195
3-pack	⅑ of 27-oz. pie	215
(Jeno's) 4-pack	¼ of 8.9-oz. pkg.	160
(Kid Cuisine)	6½-oz. pkg.	240
(Pappalo's) french bread	5.7-oz. piece	360
(Pepperidge Farm) croissant crust	1 pizza	430
(Pillsbury) microwave, regular	½ of 7.1-oz. pie	240
(Stouffer's) french bread:		
Regular, double cheese	½ of 11⅜-oz. pkg.	410
Lean Cuisine, extra cheese	5½-oz. serving	350
(Weight Watchers) regular	5⅜-oz. pie	310
Combination:		
(Jeno's) crisp 'n tasty	½ of 7.8-oz. pie	300
(Pappalo's) pan	⅙ of 26½-oz. pie	340

Food and Description	Measure or Quantity	Calories
(Pillsbury) microwave	½ of 9-oz. pie	310
(Totino's) *My Classic*, deluxe	⅙ of 22½-oz. pie	270
(Weight Watchers) deluxe	6⅜-oz. pkg.	300
Deluxe:		
(Banquet) *Zap*, french bread	4.8-oz. serving	330
(Pepperidge Farm) croissant crust	1 pizza	440
(Stouffer's) *Lean Cuisine*	6½-oz. serving	350
(Weight Watchers) french bread	6.1-oz. pkg.	310
English muffin (Empire Kosher)	2-oz. serving	140
Hamburger:		
(Fox Deluxe)	½ of 7.6-oz. pie	260
(Jeno's) 4-pack	¼ of 10-oz. pkg.	180
(Pappalo's) thin crust	⅙ of 22-oz. pie	240
(Stouffer's) french bread	½ of 12¼-oz. pkg.	410
Pepperoni:		
(Banquet) *Zap*, french bread	4½-oz. serving	350
(Fox Deluxe)	½ of 7-oz. pie	250
(Jeno's) 4-pack	¼ of 9.2-oz. pkg.	170
(Pepperidge Farm) croissant crust	1 pizza	420
(Pillsbury) microwave, regular	½ of 8½-oz. pie	300
(Totino's):		
Microwave, small	4-oz. pie	280
Party	½ of 10.2-oz. pie	370
(Weight Watchers) french bread	5¼-oz. pkg.	310
Sausage:		
(Fox Deluxe)	½ of 7.2-oz. pie	260
(Jeno's) crisp 'n tasty	½ of 7.8-oz. pie	300
(Pappalo's) pan	⅙ of 26.3-oz. pie	360
(Pillsbury) microwave, regular	½ of 8¾-oz. pie	280
(Stouffer's) french bread	½ of 12-oz. pkg.	420
(Weight Watchers)	6¼-oz. pkg.	310
Sausage & mushroom:		
(Celeste)	¼ of 24-oz. pie	365
(Stouffer's) french bread	½ of 12½-oz. pkg.	410
Sausage & pepperoni (Stouffer's) french bread	½ of 12½-oz. pkg.	450
Sicilian style (Celeste) deluxe	¼ of 26-oz. pie	408
Supreme (Celeste) without meat	½ of 8-oz. pie	217
Vegetable (Stouffer's) french bread	½ of 12¾-oz. pkg.	420
*Mix:		
(Chef Boyardee) Complete:		
Cheese	¼ of pkg.	230

Food and Description	Measure or Quantity	Calories
Pepperoni	¼ of pkg.	250
*(Ragú) *Pizza Quick*	¼ of pie	300
PIZZA PIE CRUST:		
*Mix, *Gold Medal* (General Mills)	⅙ pkg.	110
Refrigerated (Pillsbury)	⅛ of crust	90
PIZZA ROLL, frozen (Jeno's):		
Cheese	½ of 6-oz. pkg.	240
Hamburger	½ of 6-oz. pkg.	240
Sausage & pepperoni:		
Regular	½ of 6-oz. pkg.	230
Microwave	⅓ of 9-oz. pkg.	250
PIZZA SAUCE:		
(Contadina):		
Regular or with cheese	½ cup	80
With pepperoni	½ cup	90
(Ragú):		
Regular	2 oz.	32
Pizza Quick	2 oz.	45
PLUM:		
Fresh, Japanese & hybrid	2" dia.	27
Fresh, prune-type, halves	½ cup	60
Canned, regular pack:		
(Stokely-Van Camp)	½ cup	120
(Thank You Brand) heavy syrup	½ cup	109
Canned, unsweetened, purple, solids & liq.:		
(Diet Delight) juice pack	½ cup	70
(Featherweight) water pack	½ cup	40
(S&W) *Nutradiet,* juice pack	½ cup	80
PLUM JELLY, sweetened (Home Brands)	1 T.	52
PLUM PRESERVE OR JAM, sweetened (Bama)	1 T.	45
PLUM PUDDING (Richardson & Robbins)	2" wedge	270
POCKET SANDWICH, frozen:		
Lean Pockets (Chef America):		
Beef & broccoli or chicken parmesan	1 serving	250
Chicken supreme	1 serving	210
Pizza deluxe	1 serving	280
(Weight Watchers) *Ultimate 200*:		
Chicken:		
Grilled	4-oz. serving	200
Grilled, glazed	7½-oz. serving	150
Ham & cheese	4-oz. serving	200
Pizza deluxe	4-oz. serving	200

Food and Description	Measure or Quantity	Calories
POLYNESIAN-STYLE DINNER,		
frozen (Swanson)	12-oz. dinner	360
POMEGRANATE, whole	1 lb.	160
***PONDEROSA* RESTAURANT:**		
A-1 Sauce	1 tsp.	4
Beef, chopped (patty only):		
Regular	3½ oz.	209
Double Deluxe	5.9 oz.	362
Junior (*Square Shooter*)	1.6 oz.	98
Steakhouse Deluxe	2.96 oz.	181
Beverages:		
Coca-Cola	8 fl. oz.	96
Coffee	6 fl. oz.	2
Dr Pepper	8 fl. oz.	96
Milk, chocolate	8 fl. oz.	208
Orange drink	8 fl. oz.	110
Root beer	8 fl. oz.	104
Sprite	8 fl. oz.	95
Tab	8 fl. oz.	1
Bun:		
Regular	2.4-oz. bun	190
Hot dog	1 bun	108
Junior	1.4-oz. bun	118
Steakhouse deluxe	2.4-oz. bun	190
Chicken strips:		
Adult portion	2¾ oz.	282
Child	1.4 oz.	141
Cocktail sauce	1½ oz.	57
Filet mignon	3.8 oz. (edible portion)	57
Fillet of sole, fish only (See also		
Bun, regular)	3-oz. piece	125
Fish, baked	4.9-oz. serving	268
Gelatin dessert	½ cup	97
Gravy, au jus	1 oz.	3
Ham & cheese:		
Bun (See Bun, regular)		
Cheese, Swiss	2 slices (.8 oz.)	76
Ham	2½ oz.	184
Hot dog, child's, meat only (See		
also Bun, junior)	1.6-oz. hot dog	140
Margarine:		
Pat	1 tsp.	36
On potato, as served	½ oz.	100
Mustard sauce, sweet & sour	1 oz.	50
New York strip steak	6.1 oz. (edible portion)	362

Food and Description	Measure or Quantity	Calories
Onion, chopped	1 T.	4
Pickle, dill	3 slices (.7 oz.)	2
Potato:		
Baked	7.2-oz. potato	145
French fries	3-oz. serving	230
Prime ribs:		
Regular	4.2 oz. (edible portion)	286
King	6 oz. (edible portion)	409
Pudding, chocolate	4½ oz.	213
Ribeye	3.2 oz. (edible portion)	197
Ribeye & shrimp:		
Ribeye	3.2 oz.	197
Shrimp	2.2 oz.	139
Roll, kaiser	2.2-oz. roll	184
Salad bar:		
Bean sprouts	1 oz.	13
Broccoli	1 oz.	9
Cabbage, red	1 oz.	9
Carrots	1 oz.	12
Cauliflower	1 oz.	8
Celery	1 oz.	4
Chickpeas (Garbanzos)	1 oz.	102
Mushrooms	1 oz.	8
Pepper, green	1 oz.	6
Radish	1 oz.	5
Tomato	1 oz.	6
Salad dressing:		
Blue cheese	1 oz.	129
Italian, creamy	1 oz.	138
Low calorie	1 oz.	14
Oil & vinegar	1 oz.	124
1000 Island	1 oz.	117
Shrimp dinner	7 pieces (3½ oz.)	220
Sirloin:		
Regular	3.3 oz. (edible portion)	220
Super	6½ oz. (edible portion)	383
Tips	4 oz. (edible portion)	192
Steak sauce	1 oz.	23
Tartar sauce	1.5 oz.	285
T-bone	4.3 oz. (edible portion)	240

Food and Description	Measure or Quantity	Calories
Tomato (See also Salad bar):		
Slices	2 slices (.9 oz.)	5
Whole, small	3.5 oz.	22
Topping, whipped	¼ oz.	19
Worcestershire sauce	1 tsp.	4
POPCORN:		
*Home popped:		
(Jiffy Pop)	½ of 5-oz. pkg.	244
(Jolly Time) microwave:		
Natural or butter flavor	1 cup	53
Cheese flavor	1 cup	60
(Orville Reddenbacher's):		
Original:		
Plain	1 cup	22
With oil & salt	1 cup	40
Caramel crunch	1 oz.	140
Hot air popped	1 cup	25
Microwave:		
Regular:		
Butter flavored	1 cup	27
Natural	1 cup	27
Flavored:		
Caramel	1 cup	96
Cheese, cheddar	1 cup	50
Frozen	1 cup	35
(Pillsbury) microwave popcorn:		
Regular	1 cup	70
Butter flavor	1 cup	65
Pop Secret (General Mills)	1 cup	140
(Town House) microwave, natural or butter flavor	1 cup	50
Packaged:		
Buttered (Wise)	½ oz.	70
Caramel-coated:		
(Bachman)	1-oz. serving	130
(Old Dutch)	1 oz.	109
(Old London) without peanuts	1¾-oz. serving	195
(Weight Watchers)	½ oz.	60
Cheese flavored (Bachman)	1-oz. serving	180
Cracker Jack	1-oz. serving	120
(Ultra Slim Fast)	½ oz.	60
POPCORN POPPING OIL (Orville Reddenbacher's) buttery flavor	1 T.	120
***POPOVER MIX** (Flako)	1 popover	170
POPPY SEED (French's)	1 tsp.	13
***POPSICLE,** twin pop	3 fl. oz.	70

Food and Description	Measure or Quantity	Calories
POP TARTS (See TOASTER CAKE OR PASTRY)		
PORK:		
Fresh:		
Chop:		
Broiled, lean & fat	3-oz. chop (weighed without bone)	332
Broiled, lean only	3-oz. chop (weighed without bone)	230
Loin:		
Roasted, lean & fat	3 oz.	308
Roasted, lean only	3 oz.	216
Spareribs, braised	3 oz.	246
Cured ham:		
Roasted, lean & fat	3 oz.	246
Roasted, lean only	3 oz.	159
PORK, PACKAGED (Eckrich)	1-oz. serving	45
PORK, SWEET & SOUR, frozen (La Choy)	½ of 15-oz. pkg.	229
PORK DINNER OR ENTREE:		
Canned (Hunt's) *Minute Gourmet Microwave Entree Maker,* cajun:		
Without pork	3.9 oz.	180
*With pork	6.6 oz.	460
Frozen (Swanson) dinner, loin of	10¾-oz. dinner	280
PORK RINDS (Tom's)	.6 oz. serving	60
PORK STEAK, BREADED, frozen (Hormel)	3-oz. serving	223
PORT WINE:		
(Gallo)	3 fl. oz.	96
(Louis M. Martini)	3 fl. oz.	82
***POSTUM,** instant	6 fl. oz.	11
POTATO:		
Cooked:		
Au gratin	½ cup	127
Baked, peeled	2½"-dia. potato	92
Boiled, peeled	4.2-oz. potato	79
French-fried	10 pieces	156
Hash-browned, home recipe	½ cup	223
Mashed, milk & butter added	½ cup	92
Canned, solids & liq.:		
(Allen's) *Butterfield*	½ cup	45

Food and Description	Measure or Quantity	Calories
(Hunt's)	4 oz.	70
(Larsen) *Freshlike*, sliced or whole	½ cup (4.5 oz.)	61
(Town House) sliced or whole	½ cup	55
Frozen:		
(A&P)		
Regular or crinkle cut	3½-oz. serving	140
Hash brown	3½-oz. serving	80
Steak fries	3½-oz. serving	140
(Bel-Air):		
With cheese	5 oz.	220
French fries	3 oz.	120
Shoestring	3 oz.	140
With sour cream & chives	5 oz.	230
(Birds Eye):		
Cottage fries	2.8-oz. serving	119
Crinkle cuts, regular	3-oz. serving	115
Farm style wedge	3-oz. serving	109
French fries, regular	3-oz. serving	113
Hash browns, shredded	¼ of 12-oz. pkg.	61
Steak fries	3-oz. serving	109
Tasti Puffs	¼ of 10-oz. pkg.	192
Tiny Taters	⅓ of 16-oz. pkg.	204
Whole, peeled	3.2 oz.	59
(Empire Kosher) french fries	3 oz.	110
(Green Giant) one serving:		
Au gratin	5½ oz.	200
& broccoli	5½ oz.	130
(Ore-Ida):		
Cheddar Browns	3 oz.	80
Cottage fries	3 oz.	120
Crispers!	3 oz.	230
Crispy Crowns	3 oz.	170
Golden Fries	3 oz.	120
Golden Patties	3 oz.	140
Hash browns:		
Microwave	2 oz.	120
Shredded	3 oz.	70
Toaster	1¾ oz.	100
Pixie crinkles	3 oz.	140
Shoestrings	3 oz.	150
Tater Tots:		
Plain, microwave	4 oz.	200
With bacon flavor	3 oz.	150
Whole, small, seeded	3 oz.	70
(Stouffer's):		
Au gratin	⅓ pkg.	110

Food and Description	Measure or Quantity	Calories
Scalloped	⅓ pkg.	90
POTATO, STUFFED, BAKED:		
*Mix (Betty Crocker):		
Bacon & cheese	⅙ pkg.	210
Cheddar, mild, with onion	⅙ pkg.	190
Sour cream & chive	⅙ pkg.	200
Frozen:		
(Healthy Choice) with broccoli & cheese sauce	9½-oz. pkg.	240
(Oh Boy!):		
With bacon, real	6-oz. serving	116
With cheddar cheese	6-oz. serving	142
With sour cream & chives	6-oz. serving	129
(Ore-Ida):		
Butter flavor	5-oz. serving	210
Cheddar cheese	5-oz. serving	230
(Weight Watchers):		
Broccoli & cheese	10½-oz. pkg.	250
Chicken divan	11-oz. pkg.	270
POTATO & BACON, canned (Hormel) *Short Orders*, au gratin	7½-oz. can	240
POTATO & BEEF, canned, *Dinty Moore;* (Hormel) *Short Orders*	1½-oz. can	250
POTATO & HAM, canned (Hormel) *Short Orders*, scalloped	7½-oz. can	250
POTATO CHIP:		
(Cape Cod) any flavor	1 oz.	150
(Cottage Fries) unsalted	1 oz.	160
Delta Gold, any style	1 oz.	160
(Eagle):		
All types except ridged, ranch	1 oz.	150
Ridged, ranch style	1 oz.	160
(Frito-Lay):		
Natural	1 oz.	157
Ruffles, light	1 oz.	130
Sour cream & onion flavor	1 oz.	160
(Health Valley) any type	1 oz.	160
(New York Deli)	1 oz.	160
O'Grady's	1 oz.	150
(Old Dutch):		
Regular or onion & garlic	1 oz.	150
BBQ	1 oz.	140
Pringle's:		
Regular or *Cheez-Ums*	1 oz.	167
Light	1 oz.	148
(Snyder's)	1 oz.	150

Food and Description	Measure or Quantity	Calories
(Tom's) any type	1 oz.	160
(Wise):		
Barbecue or garlic & onion	1 oz.	150
Lightly salted, natural or salt & vinegar	1 oz.	160
*POTATO MIX:		
Au gratin:		
(Betty Crocker)	½ cup	150
(French's) tangy	½ cup	130
(Lipton) & sauce	¼ pkg.	108
Casserole (French's)	½ cup	130
Cheddar bacon (Lipton) & sauce	½ cup	106
Cheddar broccoli (Lipton)	½ cup	104
Chicken flavored mushroom (Lipton) & sauce	¼ pkg.	90
Hash browns (Betty Crocker) with onion	½ cup	160
Italian (Lipton)	½ cup	107
Julienne (Betty Crocker) with mild cheese sauce	½ cup	130
Mashed:		
(Betty Crocker) *Buds*	½ cup	130
(French's)	½ cup	140
(Town House)	½ cup	120
Nacho (Lipton) & sauce	½ cup	103
Scalloped:		
(Betty Crocker) plain	½ cup	140
(Libby's) *Potato Classics*	¾ cup	130
(Lipton) & sauce	¼ cup	102
*Smoky cheddar (Betty Crocker)	½ cup	140
Sour cream & chive (Betty Crocker)	½ cup	160
Stroganoff (French's) creamy	½ cup	130
*POTATO PANCAKE MIX		
(French's)	3" pancake	30
POTATO SALAD:		
Home recipe	½ cup	181
Canned (Nalley's) German style	4-oz. serving	143
*Mix (Lipton) German	½ cup	99
POTATO STICKS (Durkee) *O & C*	1½-oz. can	231
POTATO TOPPERS (Libby's)	1 T.	30
POT ROAST, frozen:		
(Armour) *Dinner Classics,* yankee	10-oz. meal	310
(Healthy Choice) yankee	11-oz. meal	260
(Le Menu) yankee	10-oz. dinner	330
(Stouffer's) *Right Course*	9¼-oz. meal	220

Food and Description	Measure or Quantity	Calories
POUND CAKE (See CAKE, Pound)		
PRESERVE OR JAM (See individual flavors)		
PRETZEL:		
(Eagle Snacks)	1 oz.	110
(Estee) unsalted	1 piece	7
Mister Salty:		
Regular:		
Dutch	.5-oz. piece	55
Logs	.1-oz. piece	12
Nuggets	1 piece	5
Rods	.5-oz. piece	55
Stick, *Veri-thin*	1 piece	2
(Rokeach)	1 oz.	110
Rold Gold	1 oz.	110
(Snyder's) hard	1 oz.	102
(Tom's) twists	1 oz.	100
(Ultra Slim Fast)	1 oz.	100
(Wise) nugget	1 oz.	110
PRODUCT 19, cereal (Kellogg's)	1 cup (1 oz.)	100
PROSCIUTTO (Hormel) boneless	1 oz.	90
PRUNE:		
Canned:		
(Featherweight) stewed, water pack	½ cup	130
(Sunsweet) stewed	½ cup	120
Dried:		
(Sunsweet) whole	2 oz.	130
(Town House)	2 oz.	140
PRUNE JUICE:		
(Algood) *Lady Betty*	6 fl. oz.	130
(Ardmore Farms)	6 fl. oz.	148
(Mott's)	6 fl. oz.	130
(Pathmark) all natural	6 fl. oz.	120
(Town House)	6 fl. oz.	120
PRUNE NECTAR, canned (Mott's)	6 fl. oz.	100
PUDDING OR PIE FILLING:		
Canned, regular pack:		
Banana:		
(Hunt's) *Snack Pack*	4¼-oz. container	180
(Thank You Brand)	½ cup	150
(Town House)	5-oz. container	160
Butterscotch:		
(Swiss Miss)	4-oz. container	160
(Thank You Brand)	½ cup	149
(Town House)	5-oz. container	160

Food and Description	Measure or Quantity	Calories
Chocolate:		
(Hunt's) *Snack Pack:*		
Regular	4¼-oz. container	160
Fudge	4¼-oz. container	170
Marshmallow	4¼-oz. container	190
(Swiss Miss) fudge or fruit on bottom	4-oz. container	170
(Thank You Brand)	½ cup	191
Rice (Comstock; Menner's)	½ of 7½-oz. can	120
Tapioca:		
(Hunt's) *Snack Pack*	4¼-oz. container	160
(Town House)	5-oz. container	160
Vanilla (Del Monte)	5-oz. container	188
Canned, dietetic pack:		
(Estee)	½ cup	70
(Sego)	4-oz. serving	125
Chilled, (Swiss Miss):		
Butterscotch, chocolate malt or vanilla	4-oz. container	150
Chocolate or double rich	4-oz. container	160
Tapioca	4-oz. container	130
Frozen (Rich's):		
Butterscotch	4½-oz. container	198
Chocolate	4½-oz. container	212
*Mix, sweetened, regular & instant:		
Banana:		
(Jell-O) cream, regular	½ cup	161
(Royal) regular	½ cup	160
Butter pecan (Jello-O) instant	½ cup	175
Butterscotch:		
(Jell-O) instant	½ cup	175
(My-T-Fine) regular	½ cup	143
Chocolate:		
(Jell-O) regular	½ cup	174
(My-T-Fine) regular	½ cup	169
Coconut:		
(Jell-O) cream, regular	½ cup	176
(Royal) instant	½ cup	170
Flan:		
(Knorr):		
Without sauce	½ cup	130
With sauce	½ cup	190
(Royal) regular	½ cup	150
Lemon:		
(Jell-O) instant	½ cup	170
(My-T-Fine) regular	½ cup	164
Lime (Royal) key lime, regular	½ cup	160

Food and Description	Measure or Quantity	Calories
Pineapple (Jell-O) cream, instant	½ cup	176
Pistachio (Jell-O) instant	½ cup	174
Raspberry (Salada) *Danish* *Dessert*	½ cup	176
Rice, (Jell-O) *Americana*	½ cup	176
Strawberry (Salada) *Danish* *Dessert*	½ cup	130
Tapioca:		
(Jell-O) *Americana,* chocolate	½ cup	173
(My-T-Fine) vanilla	½ cup	130
Vanilla:		
(Jell-O) French, regular	½ cup	172
(Royal)	½ cup	180
*Mix, dietetic:		
Butterscotch:		
(D-Zerta)	½ cup	68
(Featherweight) artificially sweetened	½ cup	60
(Royal) instant	½ cup	100
(Weight Watchers)	½ cup	90
Chocolate:		
(Estee)	½ cup	70
(Royal) instant	½ cup	100
(Weight Watchers)	½ cup	90
Vanilla:		
(D-Zerta)	½ cup	71
(Estee)	½ cup	70
(Weight Watchers)	½ cup	90
PUDDING ROLL-UPS (General Mills) *Fruit Corners*	.5-oz. roll	60
PUDDING STIX (Good Humor)	1¾-fl.-oz. pop	90
PUDDING SUNDAE (Swiss Miss):		
Caramel or mint	4-oz. container	170
Chocolate	4-oz. container	190
Peanut butter	4-oz. container	200
PUFFED RICE:		
(Malt-O-Meal)	1 cup	54
(Quaker)	1 cup	55
PUFFED WHEAT:		
(Malt-O-Meal)	1 cup	53
(Quaker)	1 cup	54
PUMPKIN, canned (Libby's) solid pack	½ cup	80
PUMPKIN BUTTER (Smucker's) *Autumn Harvest*	1 T.	36
PUMPKIN SEED, in hull	1 oz.	116

Food and Description	Measure or Quantity	Calories
PUNCH DRINK (Minute Maid):		
Canned:		
Concord, On the Go	10-fl.-oz. bottle	155
Tropical	8.45-fl.-oz. cont.	130
Chilled	6 fl. oz.	93
*Frozen, citrus	6 fl. oz.	93
PURE & LIGHT (Dole) canned:		
Country raspberry or mountain cherry	6 fl. oz.	90
Mandarin orange	6 fl. oz.	100

Food and Description	Measure or Quantity	Calories

Q

QUAIL, raw, meat & skin	4 oz.	195
QUIK, (Nestlé):		
Regular, chocolate or strawberry	1 tsp.	45
Sugar free	1 tsp.	18

Food and Description	Measure or Quantity	Calories

R

Food and Description	Measure or Quantity	Calories
RADISH	2 small radishes	4
RAISIN, dried:		
(Dole)	¼ cup	125
(Sun-Maid)	1 oz.	96
(Town House)	¼ cup	130
RAISIN SQUARES, cereal		
(Kellogg's)	½ cup	90
RALSTON, cereal (Ralston Purina)	¼ cup	90
RASPBERRY:		
Fresh:		
Black, trimmed	½ cup	49
Red, trimmed	½ cup	41
Frozen (Birds Eye) quick thaw	5-oz. serving	155
RASPBERRY DRINK, mix		
(Funny Face)	8 fl. oz.	88
RASPBERRY PRESERVE OR JAM:		
Sweetened (Smucker's)	1 T.	54
Dietetic:		
(Estee, Louis Sherry)	1 T.	6
(Slenderella)	1 T.	21
(S&W) *Nutradiet,* red	1 T.	12
RATATOUILLE, frozen (Stouffer's)	5-oz. serving	60
RAVIOLI:		
Canned, regular:		
(Franco-American) beef, *RavioliOs*	7½-oz. serving	250
(Pathmark) *No Frills,* in tomato sauce:		
Beef	7½-oz. serving	180
Cheese	7½-oz. serving	185
Canned, dietetic (Estee) beef	8-oz. can	230
Frozen:		
(Budget Gourmet) cheese:		
Regular, light	9½-oz. entree	290
Slim Selects	10-oz. meal	290
(Buitoni):		
Cheese:		
Regular, square	4.8 oz.	331

Food and Description	Measure or Quantity	Calories
Ravioletti	2.6 oz.	221
Meat, square (Celentano):	4.8 oz.	318
Regular	6½ oz.	380
Mini	4 oz.	250
(Healthy Choice) cheese, baked	9-oz. meal	250
(Kid Cuisine) cheese, mini	8¾-oz. pkg.	290
(Ultra Slim Fast) cheese	12-oz. meal	330
(Weight Watchers) baked	9 oz. meal	240
RED LOBSTER RESTAURANT: ("Lunch portion" refers to a cooked serving weighing 5 oz. raw, unless otherwise noted):		
Calamari, breaded & fried	Lunch portion	360
Catfish	Lunch portion	170
Chicken breast, skinless	4-oz. serving	140
Clam, cherrystone	Lunch portion	130
Cod, Atlantic	Lunch portion	100
Crab legs:		
King	16-oz. serving	170
Snow	16-oz. serving	150
Flounder	Lunch portion	100
Grouper	Lunch portion	110
Haddock	Lunch portion	100
Halibut	Lunch portion	110
Hamburger, without bun	5.3 oz.	320
Langostino	1 serving	120
Lobster:		
Maine	1 lobster (edible portion)	240
Rock	1 tail	230
Mackerel	Lunch portion	190
Monkfish	Lunch portion	110
Perch, Atlantic Ocean	Lunch portion	130
Pollock	Lunch portion	120
Rockfish, red	Lunch portion	90
Salmon:		
Norwegian	Lunch portion	230
Sockeye	Lunch portion	160
Scallop:		
Calico	Lunch portion	180
Deep sea	Lunch portion	130
Shark:		
Blacktip	Lunch portion	150
Mako	Lunch portion	140
Shrimp	8–12 pieces	120
Snapper, red	Lunch portion	110

Food and Description	Measure or Quantity	Calories
Sole, lemon	Lunch portion	120
Steak:		
Porterhouse	18-oz. serving	1140
Sirloin	8-oz. serving	350
Strip	9-oz. serving	560
Swordfish	Lunch portion	100
Tilefish	Lunch portion	100
Trout, rainbow	Lunch portion	170
Tuna, yellowfin	Lunch portion	180
RELISH:		
Dill (Vlasic)	1 oz.	2
Hamburger:		
(Heinz)	1 oz.	30
(Vlasic)	1 T.	24
Hot dog:		
(Heinz)	1 oz.	35
(Vlasic)	1 T.	28
India (Vlasic)	1 oz.	30
Sweet (Vlasic)	1 T.	18
RENNET MIX (Junket):		
*Powder, any flavor:		
Made with skim milk	½ cup	90
Made with whole milk	½ cup	120
Tablet	1 tablet	1
RHINE WINE:		
(Carlo Rossi)	3 fl. oz.	126
(Great Western)	3 fl. oz.	73
(Taylor)	3 fl. oz.	75
RHUBARB, cooked, sweetened	½ cup	169
***RICE:**		
Brown (Uncle Ben's) parboiled, with added butter	⅔ cup	152
White:		
(Minute Rice) instant, no added butter	⅔ cup	120
(Success) long grain	½ cooking bag	110
White & wild (Carolina)	½ cup	90
RICE, FRIED (See also RICE MIX):		
*Canned (La Choy)	⅜ cup	180
Frozen:		
(Birds Eye)	3.7-oz. serving	106
(Chun King) pork	8 oz.	270
(La Choy) & meat	8-oz. serving	280
RICE, SPANISH:		
Canned:		
Regular pack (Comstock; Menner's)	½ of 7½-oz. can	140

Food and Description	Measure or Quantity	Calories
Dietetic (Featherweight) low sodium	7½-oz. serving	140
Frozen (Birds Eye)	3.7-oz. serving	122
RICE & VEGETABLE:		
Frozen:		
(Birds Eye):		
For One:		
& broccoli, au gratin	5¾-oz. pkg.	229
Mexican, with corn	5½-oz. pkg.	158
Pilaf	5½-oz. pkg.	215
Internationals:		
Country style	3.3 oz.	87
Spanish style	3.3 oz.	111
(Budget Gourmet):		
Oriental	5¾ oz.	210
Pilaf, with green beans	5½ oz.	240
(Green Giant):		
One Serving:		
& broccoli in cheese sauce	4½-oz. pkg.	180
With peas & mushrooms with sauce	5½-oz. pkg.	130
Rice Originals:		
Medley	½ cup	100
Pilaf	½ cup	110
& wild rice	½ cup	130
*Mix:		
(Knorr) risotto	½ cup	130
(Lipton) & sauce:		
& asparagus with Hollandaise sauce	½ cup	123
& broccoli with cheddar	½ cup	131
RICE CAKE:		
(Hain):		
Regular	1 piece	40
Mini:		
Plain, apple cinnamon or teriyaki	½-oz. serving	50
Barbecue or nacho cheese	½-oz. serving	70
Cheese or honey nut	½-oz. serving	60
Heart Lovers (TKI Foods) lightly salted	.3-oz. piece	35
(Pritikin)	1 piece	35
RICE KRINKLES, cereal (Post)	⅞ cup	109
RICE KRISPIES, cereal (Kellogg's):		
Regular, frosted, cocoa or strawberry	1 oz.	110
Marshmallow	1 oz.	140

Food and Description	*Measure or Quantity*	*Calories*
RICE MIX:		
Beef:		
*(Carolina) *Bake-It-Easy*	¼ pkg.	110
(Lipton) & sauce	¼ pkg.	120
*(Minute Rice)	½ cup	149
Rice-A-Roni	⅙ pkg.	130
*Cajun (Lipton) & sauce	¼ pkg.	123
Chicken:		
*(Carolina) *Bake-It-Easy*	¼ pkg.	110
(Lipton) & sauce	¼ pkg.	125
Rice-A-Roni	⅙ pkg.	130
*Fried (Minute Rice)	½ cup	160
Herb & butter (Lipton) & sauce	¼ pkg.	124
*Long grain & wild (Minute Rice)	½ cup	150
*Milanese (Knorr) risotto, with saffron	½ cup	130
Mushroom (Lipton) & sauce	¼ pkg.	123
*Oriental (Carolina) *Bake-It-Easy*	½ pkg.	120
*Pilaf (Lipton) & sauce	½ cup	117
Spanish:		
*(Carolina) *Bake-It-Easy*	¼ pkg.	110
*(Lipton) & sauce	½ cup	120
Rice-A-Roni	⅐ pkg.	110
*Tomato (Knorr) risotto	½ cup	130
***RICE SEASONING MIX:**		
Regular (French's) *Spice Your Rice:*		
Beef flavor & onion or cheese & chives	½ cup	160
Buttery herb	½ cup	170
Fried (Kikkoman)	1-oz. pkg.	91
RICE WINE:		
Chinese, 20.7% alcohol	1 fl. oz.	38
Japanese, 10.6% alcohol	1 fl. oz.	72
RIGATONI, frozen		
(Healthy Choice) & meat sauce	9½-oz. meal	240
ROCK & RYE (Mr. Boston)	1 fl. oz.	75
ROCKY ROAD, cereal (General Mills)	⅔ cup (1 oz.)	120
ROE, baked or broiled, cod & shad	4 oz.	143
ROLL OR BUN:		
Commercial type, non-frozen:		
Apple (Dolly Madison)	2-oz. piece	180
Banquet (Mrs. Wright's)	1-oz. roll	90
Biscuit (Mrs. Wright's)	1-oz. piece	90
Blunt (Mrs. Wright's)	2-oz. piece	150
Brown & serve:		
Merita (Interstate Brands)	1-oz. roll	70

Food and Description	Measure or Quantity	Calories
(Mrs. Wright's):		
Buttermilk, gem, sesame seed or twin	1 roll	90
Half & half	1 roll	100
(Pepperidge Farm):		
Club	1 roll	100
Hearth	1 roll	50
(Roman Meal) original	1-oz. roll	72
Cherry (Dolly Madison)	2-oz. piece	180
Cinnamon (Dolly Madison)	1⅜-oz. piece	180
Club (Pepperidge Farm)	1.3-oz. piece	100
Country (Pepperidge Farm)	1 roll	50
Crescent:		
(Mrs. Wright's)	1 roll	95
(Pepperidge Farm)	1 roll	110
Croissant (Pepperidge Farm)	1 roll	170
Danish (Dolly Madison)		
Danish Twirls:		
Apple	2-oz. piece	240
Cheese, cream	3½-oz. piece	380
Cinnamon raisin	2-oz. piece	250
Dinner:		
Butternut (Interstate Brands)	1-oz. roll	90
Home Pride	1-oz. piece	85
(Mrs. Wright's) split top	1 roll	80
(Pepperidge Farm)	.7-oz. piece	60
(Roman Meal)	1-oz. roll	75
Finger (Pepperidge Farm) sesame or poppy seed	.6-oz. piece	60
Frankfurter:		
(Arnold) Hot Dog	1.3-oz. piece	100
(Mrs. Wright's) regular	1 piece	110
(Pepperidge Farm) regular	1 piece	140
(Roman Meal)	1.5-oz. roll	114
French:		
(Arnold) *Francisco,* sourdough	1.1-oz. piece	90
(Mrs. Wright) sesame	2-oz. roll	145
(Pepperidge Farm) regular	1 roll	100
Golden Twist (Pepperidge Farm)	1-oz. piece	110
Hamburger:		
(Arnold)	1.4-oz. piece	110
(Mrs. Wright's):		
Regular	2.3-oz. piece	190
Lite	1 piece	80
Onion	1 piece	130
Sesame	2.3-oz. piece	200
Wheat, crushed, giant	2.3-oz. piece	170

Food and Description	Measure or Quantity	Calories
(Pepperidge Farm) sliced	1.5-oz. piece	130
(Roman Meal)	1.6-oz. piece	122
Hoagie (Pepperidge Farm)	1 roll	210
Honey (Dolly Madison)	3½-oz. piece	420
Kaiser (Interstate Brands):		
Dutch Hearth	1½-oz. piece	110
Sweetheart	2-oz. piece	150
Lemon (Dolly Madison)	2-oz. piece	180
Old fashioned (Pepperidge Farm)	.6-oz. piece	50
Parkerhouse (Pepperidge Farm)	.6-oz. piece	60
Party (Pepperidge Farm)	.4-oz. piece	30
Potato:		
(Mrs. Wright's)	1 piece	100
(Pepperidge Farm) hearty, classic	1 piece	90
Pull-apart (Mrs. Wright's)	1 piece	170
Sandwich (Mrs. Wright's) soft	1.3-oz. roll	110
Sesame (Mrs. Wright's):		
Farmstyle	1 piece	100
Giant	2.3-oz. piece	190
Steak (Mrs. Wright's) seeded	2.5-oz. piece	220
Sub (Mrs. Wright's) junior	3-oz. piece	220
Frozen (Pepperidge Farm):		
Cinnamon	2¼-oz. piece	280
Danish:		
Apple	1 piece	220
Cinnamon raisin	1 piece	250
*ROLL OR BUN DOUGH:		
Frozen (Rich's) home style	1 piece	75
Refrigerated (Pillsbury):		
Caramel danish, with nuts	1 piece	160
Cinnamon raisin danish	1 piece	110
Crescent	1 piece	100
*ROLL MIX, HOT (Pillsbury)	1 piece	120
ROMAN MEAL CEREAL, hot:		
Regular:		
Cream of rye	⅓ cup (1.3 oz.)	112
Oat, wheat, dates, raisins, almonds	⅓ cup	136
Original, plain	⅓ cup (1 oz.)	82
Instant, oats, wheat, honey, coconut, almond	⅓ cup	154
ROSEMARY LEAVES (French's)	1 tsp.	5
ROSÉ WINE:		
Corbett Canyon (Glenmore)	3 fl. oz.	63
(Great Western)	3 fl. oz.	80

Food and Description	Measure or Quantity	Calories
(Paul Masson):		
Regular, 11.8% alcohol	3 fl. oz.	76
Light, 7.1% alcohol	3 fl. oz.	49
***ROY ROGERS* RESTAURANT:**		
Bar Burger	1 serving	573
Biscuit	1 biscuit	231
Breakfast crescent sandwich:		
Regular	4.5-oz. sandwich	408
With bacon	4.7-oz. sandwich	446
With ham	5.8-oz. sandwich	456
With sausage	5.7-oz. sandwich	564
Cheeseburger:		
Regular	1 serving	525
With bacon	1 serving	552
Chicken:		
Breast	1 piece	412
Leg	1 piece	140
Thigh	1 piece	296
Wing	1 piece	192
Chicken nugget	1 piece	48
Coleslaw	3½-oz. serving	110
Drinks:		
Coffee, black	6 fl. oz.	Tr.
Coke:		
Regular	12 fl. oz.	145
Diet	12 fl. oz.	1
Hot chocolate	6 fl. oz.	123
Milk	8 fl. oz.	150
Orange juice:		
Regular	7 fl. oz.	99
Large	10 fl. oz.	136
Shake:		
Chocolate	1 shake	358
Strawberry	1 shake	306
Vanilla	1 shake	315
Tea, iced, plain	8 fl. oz.	0
Egg & biscuit platter:		
Regular	1 meal (5.8 oz.)	557
With bacon	1 meal (6.1 oz.)	607
With ham	1 meal (7 oz.)	605
With sausage	1 meal (7.2 oz.)	713
Hamburger	1 burger	472
Pancake platter, with syrup & butter		
Plain	1 order	386
With bacon	1 order	436
With ham	1 order	434

Food and Description	Measure or Quantity	Calories
With sausage	1 order	542
Potato french fries:		
Regular	4 oz.	320
Large	5.5 oz.	440
Potato salad	3½-oz. order	107
Roast beef sandwich: Plain:		
Regular	1 sandwich	350
Large	1 sandwich	373
With cheese:		
Regular	1 sandwich	403
Large	1 sandwich	427
Salad bar:		
Bacon bits	1 T.	33
Beets, sliced	¼ cup	18
Broccoli	½ cup	12
Carrot, shredded	¼ cup	12
Cheese, cheddar	¼ cup	112
Croutons	1 T.	35
Egg, chopped	1 T.	27
Lettuce	1 cup	10
Macaroni salad	1 T.	30
Mushrooms	¼ cup	5
Noodles, Chinese	¼ cup	55
Pepper, green	1 T.	2
Potato salad	1 T.	25
Tomato	1 slice	7
Salad dressing:		
Regular:		
Bacon & tomato	1 T.	68
Bleu cheese	1 T.	75
Ranch	1 T.	77
1000 Island	1 T.	80
Low calorie, Italian	1 T.	35
Strawberry shortcake	7.2-oz. serving	447
Sundae:		
Caramel	1 sundae	293
Hot fudge	1 sundae	337
Strawberry	1 sundae	216
RUM (See DISTILLED LIQUOR)		
RUTABAGA:		
Canned (Sunshine) solids & liq.	½ cup	32
Frozen (Sunshine)	4 oz.	50

Food and Description	Measure or Quantity	Calories

S

SAFFLOWER SEED, in hull	1 oz.	89
SAGE (French's)	1 tsp.	4
SAKE WINE	1 fl. oz.	39
SALAD CRUNCHIES (Libby's)	1 T.	35
SALAD DRESSING:		
Regular:		
Bacon (Seven Seas) creamy	1 T.	60
Bacon & tomato (Henri's)	1 T.	70
Bleu or blue cheese:		
(Henri's)	1 T.	60
(Nu Made)	1 T.	60
Buttermilk (Hain)	1 T.	70
Caesar:		
(Bernstein's)	1 T.	48
(Hain)	1 T.	60
(Pfeiffer)	1 T.	70
(Wish-Bone)	1 T.	78
Capri (Seven Seas)	1 T.	70
Cheddar & bacon (Wish-Bone)	1 T.	70
Cucumber (Wish-Bone)	1 T.	80
Dijon vinaigrette (Hain)	1 T.	50
French:		
(Hain) creamy	1 T.	60
(Henri's):		
Hearty	1 T.	70
Original	1 T.	60
(Nu Made) savory	1 T.	60
(Wish-Bone) red	1 T.	64
French vinaigrette		
(Bernstein's)	1 T.	48
Garlic (Wish-Bone) creamy	1 T.	74
Garlic & sour cream (Hain)	1 T.	70
Green Goddess (Seven Seas)	1 T.	60
Honey & sesame (Hain)	1 T.	60
Italian:		
(Bernstein's) with cheese &		
garlic	1 T.	45
(Hain):		
Canola oil	1 T.	50

Food and Description	Measure or Quantity	Calories
Creamy or traditional (Henri's):	1 T.	80
Authentic	1 T.	80
Creamy garlic	1 T.	50
(Nu Made) tangy	1 T.	80
(Pfeiffer) chef	1 T.	60
(Seven Seas) *Viva!*	1 T.	70
(Wish-Bone) robusto	1 T.	70
Mayonnaise-type:		
(Luzianne Blue Plate)	1 T.	70
Miracle Whip (Kraft)	1 T.	70
Poppyseed rancher's (Hain)	1 T.	60
Ranch (Henri's) *Chef's Recipe*	1 T.	70
Red wine vinegar & oil (Seven Seas)	1 T.	60
Roquefort:		
(Bernstein's)	1 T.	65
(Marie's)	1 T.	105
Russian:		
(Henri's)	1 T.	60
(Pfeiffer)	1 T.	65
(Wish-Bone)	1 T.	45
Sour cream & bacon (Wish-Bone)	1 T.	70
Spin Blend (Hellmann's)	1 T.	57
Swiss cheese vinaigrette (Hain)	1 T.	60
Tangy citrus (Hain)	1 T.	50
Tas-Tee (Henri's)	1 T.	60
Thousand Island:		
(Bernstein's)	1 T.	62
(Nu Made)	1 T.	60
(Pfeiffer)	1 T.	65
(Wish-Bone) plain	1 T.	61
Vinaigrette (Bernstein's) french	1 T.	49
Dietetic or low calorie:		
Bleu or blue cheese:		
(Estee)	1 T.	8
(Henri's)	1 T.	35
(Tillie Lewis) *Tasti-Diet*	1 T.	12
(Wish-Bone) chunky	1 T.	40
Caesar:		
(Hain) creamy, low salt	1 T.	60
(Weight Watchers)	¾-oz. pouch	6
Catalina (Kraft)	1 T.	16
Cheese Fantastico (Bernstein's)	1 T.	15
Chef's Recipe (Henri's) ranch	1 T.	40
Cucumber (Kraft)	1 T.	30
Dijon (Estee) creamy	1 T.	8

Food and Description	Measure or Quantity	Calories
French:		
(Estee)	1 T.	4
(Henri's) original	1 T.	40
(Pritikin)	1 T.	10
(Wish-Bone) regular	1 T.	30
Garlic (Estee)	1 T.	2
Herb basket, *Herb Magic* (Luzianne Blue Plate)	1 T.	6
Italian:		
(Bernstein's) with cheese	1 T.	45
(Estee) creamy	1 T.	4
(Hain) no added salt, creamy	1 T.	80
(Henri's) hearty	1 T.	35
Herb Magic (Luzianne Blue Plate)	1 T.	4
(Pritikin) creamy	1 T.	16
(Weight Watchers) regular	1 T.	50
(Wish-Bone)	1 T.	7
Olive oil vinaigrette (Wish-Bone)	1 T.	16
Onion & chive (Wish-Bone)	1 T.	37
Ranch (Pritikin)	1 T.	18
Red wine/vinegar (Featherweight)	1 T.	6
Russian:		
(Pritikin)	1 T.	12
(Weight Watchers)	1 T.	50
(Wish-Bone)	1 T.	22
Sweet & sour, *Herb Magic* (Luzianne Blue Plate)	1 T.	18
Tas-Tee (Henri's)	1 T.	30
Thousand Island:		
(Estee)	1 T.	8
(Henri's)	1 T.	30
Herb Magic (Luzianne Blue Plate)	1 T.	8
(Kraft)	1 T.	30
(Walden Farms)	1 T.	24
(Weight Watchers)	1 T.	50
(Wish-Bone)	1 T.	36
Tomato (Pritikin) zesty	1 T.	18
2-Calorie Low Sodium (Featherweight)	1 T.	2
Vinaigrette (Pritikin)	1 T.	10
Whipped (Weight Watchers)	1 T.	45
SALAD DRESSING MIX:		
*Regular (Good Seasons):		
Blue cheese & herbs	1 T.	72

Food and Description	Measure or Quantity	Calories
Buttermilk, farm style	1 T.	58
Garlic, cheese	1 T.	72
Garlic & herb	1 T.	71
Italian, regular, cheese or zesty	1 T.	71
*Dietetic:		
Bleu cheese (Hain) no oil	1 T.	14
Buttermilk (Hain) no oil	1 T.	11
Caesar (Hain) no oil	1 T.	6
French (Hain) no oil	1 T.	12
Italian:		
(Good Seasons) lite, zesty	1 T.	26
(Hain) no oil	1 T.	2
Ranch (Good Seasons) lite	1 T.	29
1000 Island (Hain) no oil	1 T.	12
SALAD SPRAY (Richard Simmons)		
any flavor	1 spray	1
SALAD SUPREME (McCormick)	1 tsp.	11
SALAMI:		
(Eckrich) beer or cooked	1 oz.	70
Hebrew National, beef	1 oz.	80
(Hormel):		
Beef	1 slice	40
Genoa, DiLusso	1-oz. serving	100
Hard, sliced	1 slice	34
(Ohse) cooked	1 oz.	65
(Oscar Mayer):		
Beer, beef	.8-oz. slice	64
Cotto	.8-oz. slice	53
Genoa	.3-oz. slice	34
(Smok-A-Roma):		
Beef	1-oz. slice	80
Cotto	1-oz. slice	45
SALISBURY STEAK, frozen:		
(Armour) *Classics Lite*	11½-oz. meal	300
(Banquet) dinner:		
Regular	11-oz. meal	500
Extra Helping	18-oz. meal	910
(Budget Gourmet) sirloin:		
Light & Healthy	11-oz. dinner	260
Light Entree	8½-oz. entree	260
Slim Selects	9-oz. meal	260
(Healthy Choice)	11½-oz. meal	300
(Le Menu) healthy style	10-oz. dinner	280
(Morton)	10-oz. meal	300
(Stouffer's) *Lean Cuisine*	9½-oz. pkg.	280
(Swanson):		
Regular dinner, 4-compartment	10¾-oz. dinner	400

Food and Description	Measure or Quantity	Calories
Hungry Man	16½-oz. dinner	680
(Weight Watchers) beef, Romano	8¾-oz. meal	310
SALMON:		
Baked or broiled	(5.1 oz.)	264
Canned, regular pack, solids & liq.:		
Chum, *Humpty Dumpty*		
(Peter Pan) Alaska	½ cup	140
Keta (Bumble Bee)	½ cup	153
Pink or Humpback:		
(Demings) skinless & boneless	2 oz.	80
(Double "Q")	½ of 6½-oz. can	120
(Peter Pan)	½ cup	140
Sockeye or Red or Blueback:		
(Double "Q") red sockeye	½ cup	170
(Gil Netters Best) blueback	½ cup	170
Canned, dietetic (S&W) *Nutradiet*, low sodium	½ cup	188
Frozen (Captain's Choice) steak	3 oz.	183
SALMON, SMOKED (Vita):		
Lox, drained	4-oz. jar	136
Nova, drained	4-oz. can	221
SALT:		
Regular & iodized (Morton):		
Regular	1 tsp.	0
Lite	1 tsp.	0
Substitute:		
(Adolph's) plain	1 tsp.	1
Happy Heart (TKI Foods) *Just Like Salt*	⅜-oz. packet	<1
(Morton) plain	1 tsp.	Tr.
Salt-It (Estee)	1 tsp.	0
SALT 'N SPICE SEASONING		
(McCormick)	1 tsp.	3
SANDWICH SPREAD:		
(Hellmann's)	1 T.	65
(Nu Made)	1 T.	60
(Oscar Mayer)	1-oz. serving	67
SANGRIA (Taylor)	3 fl. oz.	99
SARDINE, canned:		
Atlantic (Del Monte) with tomato sauce	7½-oz. can	319
Imported (Underwood) in mustard or tomato sauce	3¾-oz. can	220
Norwegian:		
(Granadaisa Brand) in tomato sauce	3¾-oz. can	195

Food and Description	Measure or Quantity	Calories
(King David Brand) brisling in olive oil	3¾-oz. can	293
(Queen Helga Brand) in sild oil	3¾-oz. can	310
SAUCE:		
Regular:		
A-1	1 T.	12
Barbecue:		
(Heinz)	¼ cup	80
(Hunt's)	1 T.	20
(Kraft) plain or hot	¼ cup	80
(La Choy) oriental	1 T.	16
Burrito (Del Monte)	¼ cup	20
Caramel (Knorr)	1 T.	60
Cheese (Snow's) welsh rarebit	½ cup	170
Chicken Tonight (Ragú):		
Cacciatore	4 oz.	70
Country french	4 oz.	140
Creamy, with mushrooms	4 oz.	110
Herbed, with wine	4 oz.	100
Oriental	4 oz.	70
Salsa	4 oz.	35
Chili (See CHILI SAUCE)		
Cocktail:		
(Golden Dipt) regular or extra hot	1 T.	20
(Gold's)	1 T.	31
(Pfeiffer)	1-oz. serving	100
Escoffier Sauce Diable	1 T.	20
Escoffier Sauce Robert	1 T.	20
Grilling & broiling (Knorr):		
Chardonnay	⅛ pkg.	50
Spicy plum	⅛ pkg.	60
Tuscan herb	⅛ pkg.	55
Hollandaise (Knorr) microwave	1/12 pkg.	50
Hot (Gebhardt)	1 tsp.	0
Italian (See also SPAGHETTI SAUCE or TOMATO SAUCE):		
(Contadina)	4-oz. serving	71
(Ragú) red cooking	3½-oz. serving	45
Mandarin ginger (Knorr) microwave	⅛ pkg.	55
Newberg (Snow's)	⅓ cup	120
Orange (La Choy)	1 T.	23
Parmesano (Knorr) microwave	⅛ pkg.	50
Plum (La Choy) tangy	1 oz.	44
Salsa Brava (La Victoria)	1 T.	6

Food and Description	Measure or Quantity	Calories
Salsa Casero (La Victoria)	1 T.	4
Salsa Jalapeño (La Victoria)	1 T.	4
Salsa Mexicana (Contadina)	4 fl. oz.	38
Salsa Picante (La Victoria)	1 T.	4
Salsa Ranchero (La Victoria)	1 T.	6
Salsa Roja (Del Monte)	¼ cup	20
Salsa Suprema (La Victoria)	1 T.	4
Seafood cocktail (Del Monte)	1 T.	21
Soy:		
(Chun King)	1 T.	5
(Gold's)	1 T.	10
(Kikkoman) light	1 T.	13
(La Choy)	1 T.	Tr.
Spare rib (Gold's)	1 oz.	60
Sweet & sour:		
(Chun King)	1.8 oz.	57
(Contadina)	4 fl. oz.	150
(La Choy)	1 T.	30
Szechuan (La Choy)		
hot & spicy	1 oz.	48
Tabasco	¼ tsp.	Tr.
Taco:		
(La Victoria) red	1 T.	6
(Old El Paso) hot or mild	1 T.	5
(Ortega) hot or mild	1 oz.	13
Tartar:		
(Hellmann's)	1 T.	73
(Nalley's)	1 T.	89
Teriyaki (Kikkoman)	1 T.	15
V-8	1-oz. serving	25
Vera Cruz (Knorr) microwave	¼ pkg.	65
White, medium	¼ cup	103
Worcestershire:		
(French's) regular or smoky	1 T.	10
(Gold's)	1 T.	42
Dietetic:		
Barbecue (Estee)	1 T.	18
Cocktail (Estee)	1 T.	10
Mexican (Pritikin)	1 oz.	12
Soy:		
(Kikkoman)	1 T.	9
(La Choy)	1 T.	<1
Steak (Estee)	½ oz.	14
Tartar (Weight Watchers)	1 T.	35
SAUCE MIX, regular:		
À la king (Durkee)	1-oz. pkg.	133
*Au jus (Knorr)	2 fl. oz.	8

Food and Description	Measure or Quantity	Calories
*Bernaise (Knorr)	2 fl. oz.	170
*Cheese:		
(Durkee)	½ cup	168
(French's)	½ cup	160
*Demi-glace (Knorr)	2 fl. oz.	30
Hollandaise:		
(Durkee)	1-oz. pkg.	173
*(French's)	1 T.	15
*(Knorr)	2 fl. oz.	170
*Hunter (Knorr)	2 fl. oz.	25
*Italian (Knorr) Napoli	4 fl. oz.	100
*Lyonnaise (Knorr)	2 fl. oz.	20
*Mushroom (Knorr)	2 fl. oz.	60
*Pepper (Knorr)	2 fl. oz.	20
*Sweet & sour (Kikkoman)	1 T.	18
SAUERKRAUT, canned:		
(A&P)	½ cup	20
(Frank's) Bavarian	½ cup	64
(Silver Floss) solids & liq.:		
Regular	½ cup	30
Krispy Kraut	½ cup	25
(Town House)	½ cup	20
SAUSAGE:		
*Brown & Serve (Hormel)	1 sausage	70
German (Smok-A-Roma)	4-oz. link	350
Links (Ohse) hot	1 oz.	80
Patty (Hormel)	1 patty	150
Polish-style:		
(Eckrich)	1-oz. serving	95
(Hormel) *Kilbase*	1-oz. serving	122
(Ohse) regular	1 oz.	80
Pork:		
(Eckrich)	1-oz. link	100
*(Hormel) *Little Sizzlers*	1 link	51
(Jimmy Dean)	2-oz. serving	227
*(Oscar Mayer) *Little Friers*	1 link	79
Roll (Eckrich) minced	1-oz. slice	80
Smoked:		
(Eckrich) beef, *Smok-Y-Links*	.8-oz. link	70
(Hormel) smokies	1 sausage	80
(Ohse)	1 oz.	80
(Oscar Mayer) beef	1½-oz. link	126
*Turkey (Louis Rich) links or tube	1-oz. serving	45
Vienna:		
(Hormel) regular	1 sausage	50

Food and Description	Measure or Quantity	Calories
(Libby's) in barbecue sauce	2½-oz. serving	180
SAUSAGE STICK (See also BEEF JERKY):		
Beef (Pemmican):		
Pepperoni	1.1 oz.	170
Tabasco	1.1 oz.	120
Teriyaki	1.1 oz.	150
Smoked (Slim Jim):		
Big Slim	.5 oz.	80
Handi-Pak, any flavor	.3 oz.	50
Super Slim, nacho	.7 oz.	100
SAUTERNE:		
(Great Western)	3 fl. oz.	79
(Taylor)	3 fl. oz.	81
SCALLOP:		
Steamed	4-oz. serving	127
Frozen:		
(Captain's Choice) fried	1 piece	33
(Mrs. Paul's) fried, light	3 oz.	160
SCALLOP & SHRIMP DINNER, frozen (Budget Gourmet) Mariner	11½-oz. meal	410
SCHNAPPS (Mr. Boston):		
Apple	1 fl. oz.	78
Peppermint	1 fl. oz.	115
SCOTCH (See DISTILLED LIQUOR)		
SCREWDRIVER COCKTAIL (Mr. Boston) 12½% alcohol	3 fl. oz.	111
SCROD DINNER OR ENTREE, frozen (Gorton's) microwave	1 pkg.	320
SEAFOOD CREOLE, frozen (Swanson), Homestyle Recipe	9-oz. entree	240
SEGO DIET FOOD, canned:		
Regular	10-fl.-oz. can	225
Lite	10-fl.-oz. can	150
SELTZER (Canada Dry)	Any quantity	0
SERUTAN	1 tsp.	6
SESAME SEEDS (French's)	1 tsp.	9
7-ELEVEN:		
Bacon cheeseburger, *Deli-Shoppe*	6-oz. serving	558
Bagel & cream cheese, *Deli-Shoppe*	4-oz. serving	338
Big Bite:		
Regular	3.4-oz. serving	287
Super	5.4-oz. serving	460
Burrito:		
Bean & cheese	10-oz. serving	616
Beef & Bean:		

Food and Description	Measure or Quantity	Calories
Plain	5-oz. serving	308
Red chili	5-oz. serving	308
Red hot	10-oz. serving	620
Beef, bean & cheese	5.2-oz. serving	395
Chicken & rice, premium	5-oz. serving	244
Char sandwich, large, *Deli-Shoppe*	8.4-oz. serving	713
Chicken, breast of	4.8-oz. serving	405
Chimichanga, beef	5-oz. serving	363
Enchilada, beef & cheese	6½-oz. serving	369
Fajitas	5-oz. serving	311
Fish sandwich, with cheese, *Deli-Shoppe*	5.2-oz. serving	433
Sandito:		
Ham & cheese	5-oz. serving	347
Pizza	5-oz. serving	345
Sasuage, red hot, large	9.3-oz. serving	845
Tacos, twin, soft	5.9-oz. serving	399
Turkey wedge, *Deli-Shoppe*	3.4-oz. serving	193
7-GRAIN CEREAL (Loma Linda)	1 oz.	110
SHAD, CREOLE, home recipe	4-oz. serving	172
SHAKE 'N BAKE:		
Chicken:		
Original recipe	5½-oz. pkg.	617
Barbecue	7-oz. pkg.	741
Fish, original recipe	4.2-oz. pkg.	482
Pork or ribs:		
Original recipe	6-oz. pkg.	652
Extra crispy, *Oven Fry*	4.2-oz. pkg.	482
SHAKEY'S RESTAURANT:		
Chicken, fried, & potatoes:		
3-piece	1 order	947
5-piece	1 order	1700
Ham & cheese sandwich	1 sandwich	550
Pizza:		
Cheese:		
Thin	13" pizza	1403
Thick	13" pizza	1890
Onion, green pepper, olive & mushroom:		
Thin	13" pizza	1713
Thick	13" pizza	2200
Pepperoni:		
Thin	13" pizza	1833
Thick	13" pizza	2320

Food and Description	Measure or Quantity	Calories
Sausage & mushroom:		
Thin	13" pizza	1759
Thick	13" pizza	2256
Sausage & pepperoni:		
Thin	13" pizza	2111
Thick	13" pizza	2598
Special:		
Thin	13" pizza	2110
Thick	13" pizza	2597
Potatoes	15-piece order	950
Spaghetti with meat sauce & garlic bread	1 order	940
Super hot hero	1 sandwich	810
SHARK BITES (General Mills)		
Fruit Corners	.9-oz. pouch	100
SHELLS, PASTA, STUFFED, frozen:		
(Buitoni) jumbo, cheese stuffed	5½-oz. serving	288
(Celentano):		
Broccoli & cheese	13.5-oz. pkg.	540
Cheese:		
Without sauce	½ of 12½-oz. pkg.	350
With sauce	½ of 16-oz. pkg.	320
(Le Menu) healthy style	10-oz. dinner	280
(Stouffer's) cheese stuffed	9-oz. serving	320
SHERBET OR SORBET:		
Lemon (Häagen-Dazs)	4 fl. oz.	140
Lime (Lucerne)	½ cup	120
Orange:		
(Baskin-Robbins)	4 fl. oz.	158
(Borden)	½ cup	110
(Dole) mandarin	½ cup	110
(Häagen-Dazs)	4 fl. oz.	113
Peach (Dole)	½ cup	130
Pineapple (Dole)	½ cup	120
Rainbow (Baskin-Robbins)	4 fl. oz.	160
Raspberry:		
(Baskin-Robbins)	4 fl. oz.	140
(Dole)	½ cup	110
(Häagen-Dazs)	4 fl. oz.	93
(Lucerne)	½ cup	120
(Sealtest)	½ cup	140
SHERBET OR SORBET & ICE CREAM (Häagen-Dazs):		
Bar, orange & cream	1 bar	130

Food and Description	Measure or Quantity	Calories
Bulk:		
Blueberry, key lime or orange & cream	4 fl. oz.	190
Raspberry & cream	4 fl. oz.	180
SHERBET SHAKE, mix		
(Weight Watchers) orange	1 envelope	70
SHERRY:		
Cocktail (Gold Seal)	3 fl. oz.	122
Cream (Great Western) Solera	3 fl. oz.	141
Dry (Williams & Humbert)	3 fl. oz.	120
Dry Sack (Williams & Humbert)	3 fl. oz.	120
SHORTENING (See FAT, COOKING)		
SHREDDED WHEAT:		
(Kellogg's) *Squares*	½ cup (1 oz.)	90
(Nabisco):		
Regular size	¾-oz. biscuit	90
Spoon Size	⅔ cup	110
(Quaker)	1 biscuit	52
(Sunshine):		
Regular	1 biscuit	90
Bite size	⅔ cup	110
SHRIMP:		
Canned (Bumble Bee) solids & liq.	4½-oz. can	90
Frozen (Captain's Choice) cooked	3 oz.	84
SHRIMP & CHICKEN CANTONESE,		
frozen (Stouffer's) with noodles	10⅛-oz. meal	270
SHRIMP COCKTAIL canned or		
frozen (Sau-Sea)	4 oz.	113
SHRIMP DINNER, frozen:		
(Armour) *Classics Lite,* baby	9¾-oz. meal	220
(Gorton's) scampi, microwave entree	1 pkg.	470
(Healthy Choice) creole	11¼-oz. meal	210
(La Choy) *Fresh & Lite,* with lobster sauce	10-oz. meal	240
(Stouffer's) *Right Course,* primavera	9⅝-oz meal	240
(Ultra Slim Fast):		
Creole	12-oz. meal	240
Marinara	12-oz. meal	290
SLENDER (Carnation):		
Dry	1 packet	110
Liquid	10-fl.-oz. can	220
SLOPPY JOE:		
Canned:		

Food and Description	Measure or Quantity	Calories
(Hormel) *Short Orders*	7½-oz. can	340
(Libby's):		
Beef	⅓ cup	110
Pork	⅓ cup	120
Manwich (Hunt's)	1 serving	310
Frozen (Banquet) *Cookin' Bag*	5-oz. pkg.	199
SLOPPY JOE SAUCE		
(Ragú) *Joe Sauce*	3½ oz.	50
SLOPPY JOE SEASONING MIX:		
*(Durkee) pizza flavor	1¼ cups	746
(French's)	1 pkg.	128
*(Hunt's) *Manwich*	5.9-oz. serving	320
SNACK BAR (Pepperidge Farm):		
Apple nut, apricot-raspberry or		
blueberry	1.7-oz. piece	170
Brownie nut or date nut	1½-oz. piece	190
Chocolate chip or coconut		
macaroon	1½-oz. piece	210
SOAVE WINE (Antinori)	3 fl. oz.	84
SOFT DRINK:		
Sweetened:		
Apple (Slice)	6 fl. oz.	98
Birch beer (Canada Dry)	6 fl. oz.	82
Bitter lemon:		
(Canada Dry)	6 fl. oz.	75
(Schweppes)	6 fl. oz.	82
Bubble Up	6 fl. oz.	73
Cactus Cooler (Canada Dry)	6 fl. oz.	90
Cherry:		
(Canada Dry) wild	6 fl. oz.	98
(Cragmont)	6 fl. oz.	91
(Shasta) black	6 fl. oz.	81
Cherry-lime (Spree)	6 fl. oz.	79
Chocolate (Yoo-Hoo)	6 fl. oz.	93
Citrus mist (Shasta)	6 fl. oz.	85
Club	Any quantity	0
Cola:		
Coca-Cola:		
Regular or caffeine-free	6 fl. oz.	71
Classic	6 fl. oz.	61
(Cragmont) cherry	6 fl. oz.	79
Jamaica (Canada Dry)	6 fl. oz.	79
Pepsi-Cola, regular or		
Pepsi Free	6 fl. oz.	80
(Shasta) regular	6 fl. oz.	72
(Slice) cherry	6 fl. oz.	82
(Spree)	6 fl. oz.	73

Food and Description	Measure or Quantity	Calories
Collins mix (Canada Dry)	6 fl. oz.	60
Cream:		
(Canada Dry) vanilla	6 fl. oz.	97
(Schweppes)	6 fl. oz.	86
Dr. Nehi (Royal Crown)	6 fl. oz.	82
Dr Pepper	6 fl. oz.	75
Fruit punch:		
(Nehi)	6 fl. oz.	107
(Shasta)	6 fl. oz.	87
Ginger ale:		
(Canada Dry) regular	6 fl. oz.	68
(Cragmont)	6 fl. oz.	63
(Fanta)	6 fl. oz.	60
(Shasta)	6 fl. oz.	60
(Spree)	6 fl. oz.	60
Ginger beer (Schweppes)	6 fl. oz.	70
Grape:		
(Fanta)	6 fl. oz.	81
(Hi-C)	6 fl. oz.	74
(Nehi)	6 fl. oz.	96
(Schweppes)	6 fl. oz.	95
Grapefruit (Spree)	6 fl. oz.	77
Lemon lime:		
(Cragmont) cherry	6 fl. oz.	82
(Minute Maid)	6 fl. oz.	67
(Shasta)	6 fl. oz.	73
(Spree)	6 fl. oz.	77
Lemon-tangerine (Spree)	6 fl. oz.	82
Mello Yello	6 fl. oz.	87
Mountain Dew	6 fl. oz.	89
Mr. PiBB	6 fl. oz.	68
Orange:		
(Canada Dry) *Sunrise*	6 fl. oz.	68
(Cragmont)	6 fl. oz.	89
(Hi-C)	6 fl. oz.	74
(Slice)	6 fl. oz.	97
Peach (Nehi)	6 fl. oz.	102
Punch (Cragmont)	6 fl. oz.	89
Quinine or tonic water		
(Canada Dry; Schweppes)	6 fl. oz.	68
Red Pop (Shasta)	6 fl. oz.	79
Root beer:		
Barrelhead (Canada Dry)	6 fl. oz.	82
(Cragmont)	6 fl. oz.	84
(Dad's)	6 fl. oz.	83
Rooti (Canada Dry)	6 fl. oz.	82
(Shasta) draft	6 fl. oz.	77

Food and Description	Measure or Quantity	Calories
(Spree)	6 fl. oz.	77
7Up	6 fl. oz.	72
Slice	6 fl. oz.	76
Sprite	6 fl. oz.	68
Strawberry (Shasta)	6 fl. oz.	73
Tropical blend (Spree)	6 fl. oz.	73
Upper Ten (Royal Crown)	6 fl. oz.	85
Dietetic:		
Apple (Slice)	6 fl. oz.	10
Birch beer (Shasta)	6 fl. oz.	2
Bubble Up	6 fl. oz.	1
Cherry (Shasta) black	6 fl. oz.	0
Chocolate (Shasta)	6 fl. oz.	0
Coffee (No-Cal)	6 fl. oz.	1
Cola:		
(Canada Dry; Shasta)	6 fl. oz.	0
Coca-Cola, regular or caffeine free	6 fl. oz.	<1
Diet Rite	6 fl. oz.	<1
Pepsi, diet, light or caffeine free	6 fl. oz.	<1
RC	6 fl. oz.	<1
(Slice)	6 fl. oz.	10
Cream (Shasta)	6 fl. oz.	<1
Dr Pepper	6 fl. oz.	<2
Fresca	6 fl. oz.	2
Ginger ale:		
(Canada Dry)	6 fl. oz.	1
(Cragmont)	6 fl. oz.	0
(Schweppes)	6 fl. oz.	2
Grape (Shasta)	6 fl. oz.	0
Grapefruit (Shasta)	6 fl. oz.	2
Kiwi-passionfruit (Schweppes) mid-calorie royals	6 fl. oz.	35
Lemon-lime (*Diet Rite*)	6 fl. oz.	2
Mr. PiBB	6 fl. oz.	<1
Orange:		
(Canada Dry; No-Cal)	6 fl. oz.	1
(Cragmont)	6 fl. oz.	0
(Minute Maid)	6 fl. oz.	3
(Shasta)	6 fl. oz.	<1
Peach, *Diet Rite,* golden	6 fl. oz.	1
Peaches 'n cream (Schweppes) mid-calorie royals	6 fl. oz.	35
Quinine or tonic water (No-Cal)	6 fl. oz.	3
Raspberry, *Diet Rite,* red	6 fl. oz.	2
RC 100 (Royal Crown) caffeine free	6 fl. oz.	<1

Food and Description	Measure or Quantity	Calories
Red Pop (Shasta)	6 fl. oz.	0
Root beer:		
Barrelhead (Canada Dry)	6 fl. oz.	<1
(Dad's; Ramblin'; Shasta)	6 fl. oz.	<1
7Up	6 fl. oz.	2
Skipper (Cragmont)	6 fl. oz.	0
Slice	6 fl. oz.	13
Sprite	6 fl. oz.	1
Strawberry-banana (Schweppes)		
mid-calorie royals	6 fl. oz.	35
Tab, regular or caffeine free	6 fl. oz.	<1
SOLE, frozen:		
(Captain's Choice) fillet	3 oz.	99
(Frionor) *Norway Gourmet*	4-oz. fillet	60
(Healthy Choice):		
Au gratin	11-oz. meal	270
With lemon butter	8¼-oz. meal	230
(Mrs. Paul's) fillets,		
light	1 piece	240
(Van de Kamp's) batter dipped,		
french fried	1 piece	140
(Weight Watchers) stuffed	10½-oz. meal	310
SOUFFLE, frozen (Stouffer's):		
Corn	4-oz. serving	160
Spinach	4-oz. serving	140
SOUP:		
Canned, regular pack:		
*Asparagus (Campbell's),		
condensed, cream of	8-oz. serving	80
Bean:		
(Campbell's):		
Chunky, with ham,		
old fashioned	11-oz. can	290
*Condensed, with bacon	8-oz. serving	140
Home Cookin', & ham	19-oz. can	360
*(Town House) condensed, &		
bacon	8-oz. serving	140
Bean, black (Pepperidge Farm)		
with sherry	5.3-oz. serving	109
Beef:		
(Campbells):		
Chunky:		
Regular	10¾-oz. can	190
Stroganoff	10¾-oz. can	320
*Condensed:		
Regular	8-oz. serving	80
Broth	8-oz. serving	16

Food and Description	Measure or Quantity	Calories
Consommé	8-oz. serving	25
Noodle, home style	8-oz. serving	80
Home Cookin', with vegetables & pasta	19-oz. can	240
(College Inn) broth	1 cup	18
(Progresso):		
Regular	10½-oz. can	180
Hearty	½ of 19-oz. can	160
Tomato, with rotini	½ of 19-oz. can	170
Vegetable	10½-oz. can	160
(Swanson) broth	7¼-oz. can	18
Beef barley (Progresso)	10½-oz. can	170
Beef cabbage (Manischewitz)	1 cup	62
Borscht (See BORSCHT)		
*Broccoli (Campbell's) condensed, made with milk	8-oz. serving	140
Celery:		
*(Campbell's) condensed, cream of	8-oz. serving	100
*(Rokeach):		
Prepared with milk	10-oz. serving	190
Prepared with water	10-oz. serving	90
Chickarina (Progresso) plain	½ of 19-oz. can	130
Chicken:		
(Campbell's):		
Chunky:		
& rice	19-oz. can	280
vegetable	19-oz. can	340
*Condensed:		
Alphabet	8-oz. serving	80
Broth:		
Plain	8-oz. serving	30
& noodles	8-oz. serving	45
Cream of	8-oz. serving	110
Gumbo	8-oz. serving	60
Mushroom, creamy	8-oz. serving	120
Noodle:		
Regular	8-oz. serving	60
NoodleOs	8-oz. serving	70
& rice	8-oz. serving	60
Vegetable	8-oz. serving	70
Home Cookin':		
Gumbo, with sauage	10¾ oz. can	140
With noodles	19-oz. can	220
Rice	10¾ oz. can	150
(College Inn) broth	1 cup	35

Food and Description	Measure or Quantity	Calories
(Hain) broth	8¾-oz. serving	70
(Manischewitz):		
Clear	1 cup	46
Rice	1 cup	83
Vegetable	1 cup	55
(Pepperidge Farm) with wild rice	5.3-oz. serving	85
(Progresso):		
Broth	4-oz. serving	8
Cream of	½ of 19-oz. can	180
Hearty	10½-oz. can	130
(Swanson) broth, regular	7¼-oz. can	30
Chili beef (Campbell's) *Chunky*	11-oz. can	290
Chowder:		
Clam:		
Manhattan style:		
(Campbell's):		
Chunky	19-oz. can	300
*Condensed	8-oz. serving	70
(Pepperidge Farm)	5.3-oz. serving	80
(Progresso)	½ of 19-oz. can	120
*(Snow's) condensed	7½-oz. serving	70
New England style:		
*(Campbell's) condensed:		
Made with milk	8-oz. serving	150
Made with water	8-oz. serving	80
*(Gorton's)	1 can	560
(Hain)	9¼-oz. serving	180
(Pepperidge Farm)	5.3-oz. serving	133
(Progresso)	10½-oz. can	240
*(Snow's) condensed, made with milk	7½-oz. serving	140
Corn (Progresso)	½ of 18½-oz. can	200
*Fish (Snow's) condensed, made with milk	7½-oz. serving	130
Fisherman's (Pepperidge Farm) chunky	5.3-oz. serving	150
Ham'n potato (Hormel)	7½-oz. can	130
Consommé madrilene (Crosse & Blackwell)	6½-oz. serving	25
Crab (Pepperidge Farm)	5.3-oz. serving	80
Escarole (Progresso)	½ of 18½-oz. can	30
Gazpacho (Pepperidge Farm)	5.3-oz. serving	68
Ham'n butter bean (Campbell's) *Chunky*	10⅜-oz. can	280
Hunter's (Pepperidge Farm)	5.3-oz. serving	105
Italian vegetable pasta (Hain)	9½-oz. serving	160

Food and Description	Measure or Quantity	Calories
Lentil:		
(Campbell's) *Home Cookin'*	10¾ oz. can	170
(Hain) vegetarian	9½-oz. serving	160
(Progresso) with sausage	½ of 19-oz. can	180
Lobster bisque (Pepperidge Farm)	5.3-oz. serving	158
Macaroni & bean (Progresso)	10½-oz. can	180
Minestrone:		
(Campbell's):		
Chunky	19-oz. can	320
*Condensed	8-oz. serving	80
Home Cookin':		
Regular	19-oz. can	240
Chicken	19-oz. can	360
(Hain)	9½-oz. serving	170
(Pepperidge Farm)	5.3-oz. serving	110
(Progresso):		
Beef	10½-oz. can	190
Chicken	½ of 19-oz. can	130
Zesty	½ of 19-oz. can	150
*(Town House) condensed	8-oz. serving	80
Mushroom:		
*(Campbell's) condensed:		
Cream of	8-oz. serving	100
Golden	8-oz. serving	70
*(Rokeach) cream of:		
Prepared with milk	10-oz. serving	240
Prepared with water	10-oz. serving	150
*Noodle (Campbell's) & ground beef	8-oz. serving	90
*Onion (Campbell's):		
Regular	8-oz. serving	60
Cream of:		
Made with water	8-oz. serving	100
Made with water & milk	8-oz. serving	140
*Oyster stew (Campbell's):		
Made with milk	8-oz. serving	140
Made with water	8-oz. serving	70
*Pea, green (Campbell's)	8-oz. serving	160
Pea, split:		
(Campbell's):		
Chunky, with ham	19-oz. can	420
*Condensed, with ham & bacon	8-oz. serving	160
Home Cookin', with ham	10¾-oz. can	230
(Grandma Brown's)	8-oz. serving	184

Food and Description	Measure or Quantity	Calories
*Pepper pot (Campbell's)	8-oz. serving	90
*Potato (Campbell's) cream of:		
Made with water	8-oz. serving	80
Made with water & milk	8-oz. serving	120
Shav (Gold's)	8-oz. serving	25
Shrimp:		
*(Campbell's) condensed, cream of:		
Made with milk	8-oz. serving	150
Made with water	8-oz. serving	90
(Crosse & Blackwell)	6½-oz. serving	90
Steak & potato (Campbell's) *Chunky*	19-oz. can	340
Tomato:		
(Campbell's):		
Condensed:		
Regular:		
Made with milk	8-oz. serving	150
Made with water	8-oz. serving	90
& rice, old fashioned	8-oz. serving	110
Home Cookin', garden	10¾-oz. can	150
(Manischewitz)	1 cup	60
(Progresso)	½ of 19-oz. can	120
Tortellini (Progresso) regular	½ of 19-oz. can	90
Turkey (Campbell's) *Chunky*	18⅜-oz. can	300
Vegetable:		
(Campbell's):		
Chunky:		
Regular	19-oz. can	300
Beef, old fashioned	19-oz. can	320
*Condensed:		
Regular	8-oz. serving	90
Beef	8-oz. serving	70
Home Cookin':	10¾-oz. can	140
Beef	10¾-oz. can	140
Country	10¾-oz. can	120
(Hain):		
Chicken	9½-oz. serving	120
Vegetarian	9½-oz. serving	140
(Manischewitz)	1 cup	63
(Progresso)	½ of 19-oz. can	80
Vichyssoise (Pepperidge Farm)	5.3-oz. serving	114
Watercress (Pepperidge Farm)	5.3-oz. serving	90
*Won Ton (Campbell's)	8-oz. serving	40
Canned, dietetic pack:		
Bean:		

Food and Description	Measure or Quantity	Calories
*(Campbell's) condensed, *Special Request*, with bacon, less salt	8-oz. serving	140
(Pritikin) navy	½ of 14¾-oz. can	130
Beef:		
*(Campbell's) *Healthy Request*, condensed, & vegetables	8-oz. serving	70
(Healthy Choice):		
Hearty	7½-oz. serving	120
Vegetable, chunky:		
Regular	7½-oz. serving	110
Microwaveable cup	7½-oz. serving	110
(Weight Watchers) noodle	10½-oz serving	90
Beef broth:		
(Health Valley):		
Regular	7½-oz. serving	8
Fat free, no salt	6.9-oz serving	10
(Pritikin)	7¼-oz. serving	20
Chicken:		
(Campbell's):		
Regular, low sodium, with noodles	10¾-oz. can	170
Healthy Request:		
Regular, hearty, with noodles	8-oz. serving	80
*Condensed, noodle or with rice	8-oz. serving	60
Special Request, less salt:		
Cream of	8-oz. serving	110
With rice	8-oz. serving	60
(Estee) & vegetable, chunky	7¼-oz. serving	130
(Hain) broth	8¾-oz. can	60
(Health Valley):		
Fat free	6.9-oz. serving	20
Natural, no salt	7½-oz. serving	35
(Healthy Choice):		
Noodle, old fashioned	7½-oz. serving	90
Rice	7½-oz. serving	140
(Pritikin):		
Broth, defatted	½ of 13¾-oz. can	14
& ribbon pasta	½ of 14½-oz.can	60
Vegetable	½ of 14½-oz. can	70
Chowder (Pritikin):		
Manhattan	½ of 14¾-oz. can	70
New England	½ of 14¾-oz. can	118
Corn & vegetable (Health Valley) country	7½-oz. serving	70
Lentil (Pritikin)	½ of 14¾-oz. can	100

Food and Description	Measure or Quantity	Calories
*Minestrone (Estee)	7½-oz. serving	165
Mushroom (Campbell's) cream of, low sodium	10½-oz. can	210
Pea, split (Campbell's) low sodium	10¾-oz. can	230
Tomato:		
(Campbell's):		
Regular, with tomato pieces, low sodium	10½-oz. can	190
Special Request, condensed:		
Made with milk	8-oz. serving	150
Made with water	8-oz. serving	90
(Health Valley):		
Plain, natural, no salt	7½-oz. serving	130
Vegetable, fat free	7½-oz. serving	50
(Pritikin) with tomato pieces	7½-oz. serving	70
Turkey:		
(Hain) & rice, no salt added	9½-oz. serving	100
(Pritikin) vegetable	½ of 14¾-oz. can	50
(Weight Watchers) vegetable	10½-oz. can	70
Vegetable:		
(Campbell's):		
Chunky, beef, low sodium	10¾-oz. can	180
Special Request, condensed, less sodium, beef	8-oz. serving	70
(Hain) vegetarian, no salt added	9½-oz. serving	150
(Pritikin)	½ of 14⅜-oz. can	70
(Weight Watchers) vegetarian, chunky	10½-oz. can	100
Frozen:		
Asparagus (Kettle Ready) cream of	6 fl. oz.	62
*Barley & mushroom: (Empire Kosher)	7½-oz. serving	69
(Tabatchnick)	8-oz. serving	92
Bean (Kettle Ready) black	6 fl. oz.	154
Bean & barley (Tabatchnick)	8 oz.	63
Beef (Kettle Ready) vegetable	6 fl. oz.	85
Broccoli, cream of:		
(Kettle Ready) regular	6 oz.	95
(Tabatchnick)	7½ oz.	90
Cheese, cheddar (Kettle Ready)	6 oz.	158
Chicken:		
(Empire Kosher) noodle	7½-oz. serving	267

Food and Description	Measure or Quantity	Calories
(Kettle Ready):		
Cream of	6 fl. oz.	98
Gumbo	6 fl. oz.	93
Chowder:		
Clam:		
Boston (Kettle Ready)	6 oz.	131
Manhattan:		
(Kettle Ready)	6 oz.	69
(Tabatchnick)	7½ oz.	94
New England:		
(Kettle Ready)	6 oz.	116
(Stouffer's)	8 oz.	180
(Tabatchnick)	7½ oz.	97
Corn & broccoli (Kettle Ready)	6 oz.	101
Minestrone (Tabatchnick)	8 oz.	147
Mushroom (Kettle Ready) cream of	6 fl. oz.	85
Onion (Kettle Ready)	6 oz.	42
Pea, split with ham:		
(Kettle Ready)	6 oz.	155
(Tabatchnick)	8 oz.	186
Potato (Kettle Ready) cream of	8 oz.	121
Spinach, cream of:		
(Stouffer's)	8 oz.	210
(Tabatchnick)	7½ oz.	90
Tomato (Empire Kosher) florentine, cream of	6 oz.	106
Tortellini (Kettle Ready)	6 oz.	122
Vegetable:		
(Empire Kosher)	7½ oz.	111
(Kettle Ready) garden	6 oz.	85
(Tabatchnick)	8 oz.	97
*Won Ton (La Choy)	½ of 15-oz. pkg.	50
Mix, regular:		
*Asparagus (Knorr)	8 fl. oz.	80
*Barley (Knorr) country	10 fl. oz.	120
Beef:		
*(Campbell's) Cup-A-Ramen, with vegtables	8 fl. oz.	270
*(Lipton) & noodles, hearty	7 fl.oz.	107
*Broccoli (Lipton) Cup-a-Soup, creamy:		
Regular	6 fl. oz.	62
Cheese	6 fl. oz.	69
*Cauliflower (Knorr)	8 fl. oz.	100
*Cheese & broccoli (Hain)	⅜ cup	310

Food and Description	Measure or Quantity	Calories
*Chicken:		
*(Campbell's):		
Campbell's Cup, creamy	6 fl. oz.	90
Cup-A-Ramen, with		
vegetables	8 fl. oz.	270
*(Knorr)'n pasta	8 fl. oz.	90
*(Lipton):		
Regular, noodle, with		
diced white meat	8 fl. oz.	81
Cup-a-Soup:		
Regular:		
Broth	6 fl. oz.	19
Cream of	6 fl. oz.	84
& rice	6 fl. oz.	47
Hearty:		
Country style	6 fl. oz.	69
& noodles	6 fl. oz.	110
Lots-A-Noodles, creamy,		
hearty	7 fl. oz.	179
*Chowder (Gorton's) New		
England	¼ of can	140
*Herb (Knorr) fine	8 fl. oz.	130
*Hot & sour (Knorr)	8 fl. oz.	80
*Leek (Knorr)	8 fl. oz.	110
*Lentil (Hain) savory	¾ cup	130
*Minestrone:		
(Hain)	¾ cup	110
(Knorr) hearty	10 fl. oz.	130
(Manischewitz)	6 fl. oz.	50
*Mushroom:		
*(Knorr)	8 fl. oz.	100
(Lipton):		
Regular, beef	8 fl. oz.	38
Cup-a-Noodles, cream of	6 fl. oz.	70
*Noodle:		
(Campbell's):		
(*Campbell's Cup*):		
Regular, with chicken		
broth	6 fl. oz.	90
Microwavable cup:		
Beef flavor	1 cup	130
Hearty	1 cup	180
Quality soup & recipe:		
Regular	8 fl. oz.	110
Hearty	8 fl. oz.	90
Ramen:		
Beef flavor	8 fl. oz.	190

Food and Description	Measure or Quantity	Calories
Pork flavor	8 fl. oz.	50
(4C)	8 fl. oz.	50
*Onion:		
*(Hain)	¾ cup	50
*(Knorr) french	8 fl. oz.	50
(Lipton):		
Regular, beef	8 fl. oz.	24
Cup-a-Soup	6 fl. oz.	27
*Oriental (Campbell's) *Cup-A-Ramen*	8 fl. oz.	270
*Oxtail (Knorr) hearty beef	8 fl. oz.	70
*Pea, green (Lipton) *Cup-a-Soup*	6 fl. oz.	113
*Pea, split (Hain)	¾ cup	310
*Tomato (Lipton) *Cup-a-Soup*	6 fl. oz.	103
*Tomato onion (Lipton)	8 fl. oz.	80
*Tortellini (Knorr)	8 fl. oz.	60
*Vegetable:		
(Campbell's) quality soup	8 fl.oz.	40
(Hain)	¾ cup	80
(Knorr) spring, with herbs	8 fl. oz.	30
(Lipton):		
Regular, country	8 fl. oz.	80
Cup-a-Soup:		
Regular, spring	6 fl. oz.	41
Country style, harvest	6 fl. oz.	94
Lots-A-Noodles, garden	7 fl. oz.	123
(Manischewitz)	6 fl. oz.	50
(Southland) frozen	⅕ of 16-oz. pkg.	60
Mix, dietetic:		
Beef:		
*(Estee) noodle	6 fl. oz.	20
(Weight Watchers) broth	1 packet	8
*Broccoli (Lipton) *Cup-a-Soup,* lite, golden	6 fl. oz.	42
Chicken:		
*(Lipton) *Cup-a-Soup,* lite:		
Florentine	6 fl. oz.	42
Lemon	6 fl. oz.	48
(Weight Watchers) broth	1 packet	8
*Mushroom:		
(Estee) cream of	6 fl. oz.	40
(Hain) no added salt	⅜ cup	250
*Noodle (Campbell's) ramen, low fat block:		
Beef flavor	8 fl. oz.	160
Pork flavor	8 fl. oz.	150
*Onion:		

Food and Description	Measure or Quantity	Calories
(Estee)	6 fl. oz.	25
(4C) reduced salt	8 fl. oz.	30
(Hain) no salt added	3/8 cup	50
*Oriental:		
(Campbell's) *Cup-A-Ramen*	8 fl. oz.	220
(Lipton) *Cup-a-Soup*, lite	6 fl. oz.	45
*Shrimp (Campbell's) *Cup-A-Ramen*,		
with vegetables, low fat	8 fl. oz.	230
*Tomato:		
(Estee)	6 fl. oz.	40
(Lipton) *Cup-a-Soup*, lite, herb	6 fl. oz.	65
SOUP GREENS (Durkee)	2⅓-oz. jar	216
SOUTHERN COMFORT:		
80 proof	1 fl. oz.	79
100 proof	1 fl. oz.	95
SOYBEAN CURD OR TOFU	2¾" × 1½" × 1" cake	86
SOYBEAN OR NUT:		
Dry roasted (*Soy Ahoy; Soy Town*)	1 oz.	139
Oil roasted (*Soy Ahoy; Soy Town*)		
plain, barbecue or garlic	1 oz.	152
SPAGHETTI:		
Dry (Pritikin) whole wheat	1 oz.	110
Cooked:		
8-10 minutes, "Al Dente"	1 cup	216
14-20 minutes, tender	1 cup	155
Canned:		
(Franco-American):		
tomato sauce	7⅜-oz. can	220
With meatballs in tomato sauce, *SpaghettiOs*	7⅜-oz. can	220
With sliced franks in tomato sauce, *SpaghettiOs*	7⅜-oz. can	210
(Hormel) *Short Orders*, & meatballs in tomato sauce	7½-oz. can	210
(Libby's) & meatballs in tomato sauce	7½-oz. serving	189
Dietetic (Estee) & meatballs	7½-oz. serving	240
Frozen:		
(Armour) *Dining Lite*, with meat	9-oz. meal	220
(Banquet) & meat sauce	8-oz. pkg.	270
(Le Menu) healthy style	9-oz. entree	280
(Morton) & meatball	10-oz. dinner	200
(Stouffer's) *Lean Cuisine*	11½-oz. pkg.	280

Food and Description	Measure or Quantity	Calories
(Swanson):		
Regular, & meatballs	12½-oz. dinner	390
Homestyle Recipe	13-oz. entree	490
(Weight Watchers) with meat sauce	10½-oz. meal	280
SPAGHETTI SAUCE, canned:		
Regular pack:		
Alfredo (Progresso), seafood	½ cup	220
Bolognese (Progresso)	½ cup	150
Cheese (Prego)	4-oz. serving	100
Chunky (Hunt's)	4-oz. serving	50
Clam (Progresso) white, authentic pasta sauce	½ cup	130
Garden Style (Ragú)	4-oz. serving	80
Homestyle (Hunt's)	4 oz.	60
Lobster (Progresso) rock	½ cup	120
Marinara:		
(Prince)	4-oz. serving	80
(Progresso):		
Regular	½ cup	90
Authentic pasta sauce	½ cup	110
(Ragú)	5-oz. serving	120
Meat or meat flavored:		
(Hunt's)	4-oz. serving	70
(Prego)	4-oz. serving	140
(Ragú) regular	4-oz. serving	80
(Town House)	4-oz. serving	80
Meatless or plain:		
(Prego)	4-oz. serving	140
(Ragú) regular	4-oz. serving	80
(Town House)	4-oz. serving	80
Mushroom:		
(Hain)	4-oz. serving	80
(Hunt's) regular	4-oz. serving	70
(Prego) regular	4-oz. serving	130
(Progresso)	½ cup	110
(Ragú) Extra Thick & Zesty	4-oz. serving	110
Primavera (Progresso) creamy	½ cup	190
Romano (Progresso) creamy	½ cup	220
Sausage & green pepper (Prego)	4-oz. serving	160
Seafood (Progresso):		
Regular	½ cup	110
Authentic pasta sauce	½ cup	190
Sicilian (Progresso)	½ cup	30
Tomato & basil (Prego)	4-oz. serving	100

Food and Description	Measure or Quantity	Calories
Traditional (Hunt's)	4 oz. serving	70
Veal (Prego Plus)	4-oz. serving	150
Dietetic pack:		
(Estee)	4-oz. serving	60
(Furman's) low sodium	½ cup	83
(Prego) low sodium	½ cup	110
(Pritikin) plain or mushroom	4-oz. serving	60
(Weight Watchers) mushroom	⅓ cup	40
SPAGHETTI SAUCE MIX:		
*(Durkee) regular	½ cup	45
*(French's) with mushrooms	⅝ cup	100
(Lawry's) rich & thick	1½-oz. pkg.	147
*(Spatini)	½ cup	84
***SPAM,** luncheon meat (Hormel):*		
Regular, smoke flavored or with cheese chunks	1-oz. serving	85
Deviled	1 T.	35
SPARKLING COOLER CITRUS,		
La Croix (Heilemann)	6 fl. oz.	107
***SPECIAL K,** cereal (Kellogg's)*	1 cup (1 oz.)	110
SPINACH:		
Fresh, whole leaves	½ cup	4
Boiled	½ cup	18
Canned, regular pack (Allen's) solids & liq.	½ cup	25
Canned, dietetic pack (Del Monte) no salt added	½ cup	25
Frozen:		
(A&P) leaf	3.3 oz.	25
(Bel-Air)	3.3 oz.	20
(Birds Eye):		
Chopped or leaf	⅓ pkg.	28
Creamed	⅓ pkg.	60
(Budget Gourmet) au gratin	6 oz.	120
(Green Giant):		
Creamed	3.3 oz.	40
Harvest Fresh	4.5 oz. serving	25
SPINACH PUREE, canned		
(Larsen) low sodium	½ cup	22
SQUASH, SUMMER:		
Fresh, yellow, boiled slices	½ cup	13
Fresh, zucchini, boiled slices	½ cup	9
Canned (Progresso) zucchini, in tomato sauce	½ cup	50
Frozen:		
(Birds Eye) zucchini	⅓ pkg.	19
(Larsen) yellow crookneck	3.3 oz.	18

Food and Description	Measure or Quantity	Calories
(McKenzie) crookneck	⅓ pkg.	20
(Mrs. Paul's) sticks, batter dipped, french fried	⅓ pkg.	180
(Ore-Ida) breaded	3 oz.	150
SQUASH, WINTER:		
Acorn, baked	½ cup	56
Hubbard, baked, mashed	½ cup	51
Frozen:		
(Birds Eye)	⅓ pkg.	43
(Southland) butternut	4-oz. serving	45
STEAK (See BEEF)		
STEAK & GREEN PEPPERS:		
Frozen:		
(Green Giant)	9-oz. entree	250
(Swanson)	8½-oz. entree	200
STEAK UMM	2 oz.	180
STOCK BASE (French's) beef or chicken	1 tsp.	8
STRAWBERRY:		
Fresh, capped	½ cup	26
Frozen (Birds Eye):		
Halves	⅓ pkg.	164
Whole	¼ pkg.	89
Whole, quick thaw	½ pkg.	125
STRAWBERRY FRUIT JUICE, canned (Smucker's)	8 fl. oz.	120
STRAWBERRY NECTAR, canned (Libby's)	6 fl. oz.	60
STRAWBERRY PRESERVE OR JAM:		
Sweetened:		
(Bama)	1 T.	45
(Smucker's)	1 T.	53
(Welch's)	1 T.	52
Dietetic or low calorie:		
(Estee; Louis Sherry)	1 T.	6
(Diet Delight)	1 T.	12
(Featherweight) calorie reduced	1 T.	16
STUFFING, frozen (Green Giant)		
Stuffing Originals:		
Chicken or cornbread	½ cup	170
Mushroom	½ cup	150
Wild rice	½ cup	160
STUFFING MIX:		
Apple & raisin (Pepperidge Farm)	1 oz.	110
*Beef, Stove Top	½ cup	180

Food and Description	Measure or Quantity	Calories
*Chicken:		
*(Bell's)	½ cup	224
*(Betty Crocker)	⅕ pkg.	180
Stove Top	½ cup	180
*Cornbread, Stove Top	½ cup	170
Cube or herb seasoned (Pepperidge Farm)	1 oz.	110
*Herb (Betty Crocker) traditional	⅙ pkg.	190
*Pork, Stove Top	½ cup	170
*Premium Blend (Bell's)	½ cup	180
*Ready Mix (Bell's)	½ cup	224
White bread (Mrs. Cubbison's)	1 oz.	101
STURGEON, smoked	4-oz. serving	169
SUCCOTASH:		
Canned:		
(Comstock) whole kernel	½ cup	80
(Larsen) Freshlike	½ cup	80
(Libby's) cream style	½ cup	111
(Stokely-Van Camp)	½ cup	85
Frozen:		
(Bel-Air)	3.3 oz.	100
(Birds Eye)	⅓ pkg.	104
(Frosty Acres)	3.3 oz.	100
***SUDDENLY SALADS** (General Mills):		
Macaroni, creamy	⅙ pkg.	200
Pasta, Italian	⅙ pkg.	160
Potato, creamy	⅙ pkg.	250
SUGAR:		
Brown, dark or light	1 T.	48
Confectioners	1 T.	30
Granulated	1 T.	46
Maple	1¾" × 1¼" × ½" piece	104
SUGAR SUBSTITUTE:		
(Estee)	1 tsp.	12
(Featherweight)	3 drops	0
(Pritikin) Supreme	1.76-oz. packet	3
Sprinkle Sweet (Pillsbury)	1 tsp.	2
Sweet'n-it (Estee) liquid	5 drops	0
Sweet 'N Low:		
Brown	1 tsp.	20
Granulated	1-gram packet	4
Liquid	1 drop	0
***SUGAR PUFFS,** cereal (Malt-O-Meal)	⅞ cup	110

Food and Description	Measure or Quantity	Calories
*SUKIYAKI DINNER (Chun King) stir fry	6 oz.	257
SUNFLOWER SEED (Fisher):		
In hull, roasted, salted	1 oz.	86
Hulled, dry roasted, salted	1 oz.	164
Hulled, oil roasted, salted	1 oz.	167
SUNTOPS (Dole)	1 bar	40
SURIMI (See CRAB SUBSTITUTE)		
SWEETBREADS, calf, braised	4-oz. serving	191
SWEET POTATO:		
Baked, peeled	5" × 1" potato	155
Canned:		
(Allen's)	4-oz. serving	50
(Joan of Arc):		
Mashed	½ cup	90
Whole:		
Candied	½ cup	240
Heavy syrup	½ cup	130
In pineapple-orange sauce	½ cup	210
(Trappey's) *Sugary Sam:*		
Cut	½ cup (4.3 oz.)	110
Whole	½ cup (4.3 oz.)	130
Frozen:		
(Mrs. Paul's) candied, with apples	4-oz. serving	160
(Stouffer's) & apples	5-oz. serving	160
SWEET 'N SOUR COCKTAIL MIX (Holland House) liquid	1 fl. oz.	34
SWEET & SOUR PORK, frozen:		
(Chun King)	13-oz. entree	400
(La Choy)	12-oz. entree	360
SWISS STEAK, frozen (Swanson)	10-oz. dinner	350
SWORDFISH:		
Broiled	3"× 3" × ½" steak	218
Frozen (Captain's Choice) steak	3 oz.	132
SYRUP (See also TOPPING):		
Regular:		
Blackberry (Smucker's)	1 T.	50
Boysenberry (Smucker's)	1 T.	50
Chocolate or chocolate-flavored:		
Bosco	1 T.	55
(Hershey's)	1 T.	40
(Nestlé) *Quik*	1 oz.	80
Corn, *Karo,* dark or light	1 T.	60
Maple, *Karo,* imitation	1 T.	57

Food and Description	Measure or Quantity	Calories
Pancake or waffle:		
(Aunt Jemima)	1 T.	53
(Glencourt) *Piedmont*, old fashioned	1 T.	50
Golden Griddle	1 T.	54
Karo	1 T.	58
Log Cabin, regular or buttered	1 T.	72
Mrs. Butterworth's	1 T.	55
(Smucker's)	1-oz. packet	116
Strawberry (Smucker's)	1 T.	50
Dietetic or low calorie:		
Blueberry (Estee)	1 T.	4
Chocolate or chocolate-flavored (Estee)	1 T.	20
Maple (S&W) *Nutradiet*	1 T.	12
Pancake or waffle:		
(Aunt Jemima)	1 T.	29
(Cary's)	1 T.	6
(Estee)	1 T.	8
Log Cabin	1 T.	34
(Weight Watchers)	1 T.	25

Food and Description	Measure or Quantity	Calories

T

TACO:
*(Ortega)	1 oz.	54
*Mix (Durkee)	½ cup	321
Shell (Ortega)	1 shell	50

***TACO BELL* RESTAURANT:**

Burrito:

Bean:
Green sauce	6¾-oz. serving	351
Red sauce	6¾-oz. serving	357

Beef:
Green sauce	6¾-oz. serving	398
Red sauce	6¾-oz. serving	403

Supreme:

Regular:
Green sauce	8½-oz. serving	407
Red sauce	8½-oz. serving	413

Double beef:
Green sauce	9-oz. serving	451
Red sauce	9-oz. serving	456

Cinnamon crispas	1.7-oz. serving	259

Enchirito:
Green sauce	7½-oz. serving	371
Red sauce	7½-oz. serving	382

Fajita:
Chicken	4¾-oz. serving	225
Steak	4¾-oz. serving	234
Guacamole	¾-oz. serving	34
Meximelt	3¾-oz. serving	266

Nachos:
Regular	3¾-oz. serving	345
Bellgrande	10.1-oz. serving	648
Pepper, jalapeño	3½-oz. serving	20
Pico De Gallo	1-oz. serving	8

Pintos & cheese:
Green sauce	4½-oz. serving	184
Red sauce	4½-oz. serving	190
Pizza, Mexican	7.9-oz. serving	575
Ranch dressing	2.6-oz. serving	235
Salsa	.3-oz. serving	18

Food and Description	Measure or Quantity	Calories
Sour cream	¾-oz. serving	46
Taco:		
Regular	2¾-oz. serving	183
Bellgrande	5¾-oz. serving	355
Light	6-oz. serving	410
Soft:		
Regular	3¼-oz. serving	338
Supreme	4.4-oz. serving	275
Super combo	5-oz. serving	286
Taco salad:		
With shell	18.7-oz. serving	502
With salsa:		
Regular	21-oz. serving	941
Without shell	18.7-oz. serving	520
Taco sauce:		
Regular	.4-oz. packet	2
Hot	.4-oz. packet	2
Tostada:		
Green sauce	5½-oz. serving	237
Red sauce	5½-oz. serving	243

TACO JOHN'S RESTAURANT:

Food and Description	Measure or Quantity	Calories
Burrito:		
Bean	5-oz. serving	197
Beef	5-oz. serving	303
Chicken:		
Regular	5-oz. serving	227
With green chili	12¼-oz. serving	344
Combo	5-oz. serving	250
Smothered:		
With green chili	12¼-oz. serving	367
With Texas chili	12¼-oz. serving	455
Super:		
Regular	8¼-oz. serving	389
With chicken	8¼-oz. serving	366
Chimichanga:		
Regular	12-oz. serving	464
With chicken	12-oz. serving	441
Mexican rice	8-oz. serving	340
Nachos:		
Regular	5-oz. serving	468
Super	11¼-oz. serving	669
Potato Ole, large	6-oz. serving	414
Taco:		
Regular	4¼-oz. serving	178
With chicken	4¼-oz. serving	140
Soft shell:		
Regular	5-oz. serving	224

Food and Description	Measure or Quantity	Calories
With chicken	5-oz. serving	180
Taco Bravo:		
Regular	6¾-oz. serving	319
Super	8-oz. serving	361
Taco burger	6-oz. serving	281
Taco salad:		
Regular:		
Without dressing	6-oz. serving	229
With dressing	8-oz. serving	359
Chicken:		
Without dressing	12¼-oz. serving	377
With dressing	14¼-oz. serving	507
Super:		
Without dressing	12¼-oz. serving	428
With dressing	14¼-oz. serving	558
TAMALE:		
Canned:		
(Hormel) beef, *Short Orders*	7½-oz. can	270
(Old El Paso)	1 tamale	95
(Pride of Mexico) beef	1 tamale	115
Frozen (Hormel) beef	1 tamale	130
TANG:		
Canned, *Fruit Box:*		
Cherry or strawberry	8.45-fl.-oz. container	121
Grape	8.45-fl.-oz. container	131
Mixed fruit	8.45-fl.-oz. container	137
Orange, regular	8.45-fl.-oz. container	127
*Mix:		
Regular	6 fl. oz.	86
Dietetic	6 fl. oz.	5
TANGERINE OR MANDARIN ORANGE:		
Fresh (Sunkist)	1 large tangerine	39
Canned, solids & liq.:		
Regular pack (Dole)	½ cup	70
Dietetic pack:		
(Diet Delight) juice pack	½ cup	50
(Featherweight) water pack	½ cup	35
(S&W) *Nutradiet*	½ cup	28
TANGERINE DRINK, canned (Hi-C)	6 fl. oz.	90
TANGERINE JUICE, frozen (Minute Maid)	6 fl. oz.	91
TAPIOCA, dry, *Minute,* quick cooking	1 T.	32
TAQUITO, frozen (Van de Kamp's) beef	8-oz. serving	490

Food and Description	Measure or Quantity	Calories
TARRAGON (French's)	1 tsp.	5
TASTEEOS, cereal (Ralston Purina)	1¼ cups (1 oz.)	110
***TEA:**		
Bag:		
(Celestial Seasonings):		
After dinner:		
Amaretto Nights or *Swiss Mint*	1 cup	<3
Bavarian Chocolate Orange	1 cup	7
Caffeine free	1 cup	4
Fruit & tea	1 cup	<3
Herb:		
Almond Sunset, Cinnamon Apple or *Cranberry Cove*	1 cup	3
Emperor's Choice or *Lemon Zinger*	1 cup	4
Mandarin Orange Spice or *Orange Zinger*	1 cup	5
Roastaroma	1 cup	11
Premium black tea	1 cup	3
(Lipton):		
Plain or flavored	1 cup	2
Herbal:		
Almond Pleasure or *Cinnamon Apple*	1 cup	2
Quietly Chamomile or *Toasty Spice*	1 cup	6
(Sahadi) spearmint	1 cup	4
Instant (Nestea)100%	6 fl. oz.	0
TEA MIX, ICED:		
*(4C)	8 fl. oz.	90
*(Lipton) lemon & sugar flavored	1 cup	60
Nestea, lemon-flavored	1 cup	6
*Dietetic, *Crystal Light*	8 fl. oz.	3
TEMPURA BATTER, mix (Golden Dipt)	1 oz.	100
TEQUILA SUNRISE COCKTAIL,		
(Mr. Boston) 12½% alcohol	3 fl. oz.	120
TERIYAKI:		
*Canned (La Choy) chicken	⅜ cup	85
Frozen:		
(Chun King)	13-oz. entree	380
(La Choy) *Fresh & Lite*	10-oz. meal	240
(Stouffer's) beef	9⅜-oz. serving	290
TERIYAKI BASTE & GLAZE		
(Kikkoman)	1 T.	24

Food and Description	Measure or Quantity	Calories
*TEXTURED VEGETABLE PROTEIN,		
Morningstar Farms:		
Breakfast link	1 link	73
Breakfast patties	1 patty	100
Breakfast strips	1 strip	37
Grillers	1 patty	190
THURINGER:		
(Eckrich) *Smoky Tang*	1-oz. serving	80
(Hormel):		
Beefy	1-oz. serving	100
Old Smokehouse	1-oz. serving	100
(Louis Rich) turkey	1-oz. serving	50
(Ohse) beef	1 oz.	80
(Oscar Mayer) beef	.8-oz. slice	69
TOASTER CAKE OR PASTRY:		
Pop-Tarts (Kellogg's):		
Regular:		
Blueberry, brown sugar, cinnamon or cherry	1 pastry	210
Strawberry	1 pastry	200
Frosted:		
Blueberry, chocolate fudge or strawberry	1 pastry	200
Brown sugar cinnamon, cherry	1 pastry	210
Toaster Strudel (Pillsbury)	1 slice	190
Toaster Tarts (Pepperidge Farm):		
Apple cinnamon	1 piece	170
Strawberry	1 piece	190
Toastettes (Nabisco) regular or frosted	1 piece	200
Toast-R-Cake (Thomas'):		
Blueberry	1 piece	108
Bran	1 piece	103
Corn	1 piece	120
TOASTY O'S, cereal (Malt-O-Meal)	1¼ cup	107
TOFUTTI:		
Frozen:		
Regular:		
Chocolate supreme or wildberry supreme	4 fl. oz.	210
Maple walnut	4 fl. oz.	230
Vanilla	4 fl. oz.	200
Cuties:		
Chocolate	1 piece	140
Vanilla	1 piece	130

Food and Description	Measure or Quantity	Calories
Lite Lite	4 fl. oz.	90
Love Drops: Cappuccino or chocolate	4 fl. oz.	230
Vanilla	4 fl. oz.	220
Soft serve:		
Regular	4 fl. oz.	158
Hi-Lite:		
Chocolate	4 fl. oz.	100
Vanilla	4 fl. oz.	90
TOMATO:		
Regular, whole	1 med. tomato	33
Cherry, whole	4 pieces	14
Canned, regular pack, solids & liq.:		
Angela Mia (Hunt's) crushed	4 oz.	35
(Contadina) sliced, baby	½ cup	50
(Hunt's):		
Crushed, Italian	½ cup	40
Pear shaped, Italian	4 oz.	20
Stewed, regular	½ cup (4 oz.)	35
Whole, regular	4 oz.	20
(La Victoria) green, whole	1 oz.	8
(Pathmark) No Frills, crushed	½ cup	45
(Town House) stewed	½ cup	35
Canned, dietetic pack, solids & liq.:		
(Del Monte) No Salt Added	½ cup	35
(Featherweight)	½ cup	20
(Furman's) low sodium	½ cup	72
(Hunt's) whole	4 oz.	20
(Pathmark) whole, seeded, no salt added	½ cup	25
TOMATO, PICKLED (Claussen) green	1 piece	6
TOMATO & PEPPER, HOT CHILI, (Old El Paso) Jalapeño	¼ cup	13
TOMATO JUICE, canned:		
Regular pack:		
(A&P)	6 fl. oz.	30
(Ardmore Farms)	6-fl.-oz. can	36
(Campbell's)	6-fl.-oz. can	40
(Hunt's)	6 fl. oz.	30
(Pathmark)	6 fl. oz.	30
(Town House)	6 fl. oz.	35
Dietetic pack (Diet Delight; Featherweight)	6 fl. oz.	35
TOMATO JUICE COCKTAIL, canned:		
(Ocean Spray) Firehouse Jubilee	6 fl. oz.	44

Food and Description	Measure or Quantity	Calories
SnapE-Tom	6 fl. oz.	40
TOMATO PASTE, canned:		
Regular pack:		
(A&P)	6-oz. serving	150
(Contadina) Italian	6-oz. serving	210
(Hunt's) Italian style	6 oz.	150
(Pathmark) California	⅔ cup	150
Dietetic (Hunt's) low sodium	6-oz. can	135
TOMATO PUREE, canned:		
Regular (Contadina) heavy	1 cup	100
Dietetic (Featherweight)	1 cup	90
TOMATO SAUCE, canned:		
(A&P)	½ cup	45
(Del Monte):		
Regular or no salt added	1 cup	70
Hot	½ cup	40
With tomato bits	1 cup	92
(Furman's)	½ cup	58
(Hunt's):		
Regular or with bits	4 oz.	30
With garlic	4 oz.	70
(Pathmark)	½ cup	40
(Town House)	4 oz.	40
TOM COLLINS (Mr. Boston)		
12½% alcohol	3 fl. oz.	111
*TOM COLLINS MIX,		
(Bar-Tender's)	6 fl. oz.	177
TONGUE, beef, braised	4-oz. serving	277
TOPPING:		
Regular:		
Butterscotch (Smucker's)	1 T.	70
Caramel (Smucker's) regular	1 T.	70
Chocolate fudge (Hershey's)	1 T.	50
Fudge, hot (Smucker's) special recipe	1 T.	75
Marshmallow (Smucker's)	1 T.	60
Pecans in syrup (Smucker's)	1 T.	65
Pineapple (Smucker's)	1 T.	65
Strawberry (Smucker's)	1 T.	60
Walnuts in syrup (Smucker's)	1 T.	65
Dietetic, chocolate (Smucker's)	1 T.	35
TOPPING, WHIPPED:		
Regular:		
Cool Whip (Birds Eye) dairy	1 T.	16
(Johanna Farms) aerosol	1 T.	8
Lucky Whip, aerosol	1 T.	12
(Party Whip) non-dairy	1 T.	10

Food and Description	Measure or Quantity	Calories
Dietetic (Featherweight)	1 T.	3
*Mix:		
Regular, *Dream Whip*	1 T.	5
Dietetic (D-Zerta; Estee)	1 T.	4
TOP RAMEN, beef (Nissin Foods)	3-oz. serving	390
TORTELLINI, frozen:		
(Budget Gourmet) cheese	5½-oz. pkg.	180
(Buitoni):		
Cheese filled, verdi	2.6-oz. serving	220
Meat filled	2.5-oz. entree	223
(Green Giant) cheese marinara, One Serving	5½-oz. pkg.	260
(Le Menu) cheese, healthy style, with meat sauce	8-oz. entree	250
(Stouffer's):		
Cheese filled, with tomato sauce	9⅝-oz. meal	360
Veal stuffed, in Alfredo sauce	8⅝-oz. meal	500
TORTILLA (Amigos)	6" × ⅛" tortilla	111
TOSTADA, frozen (Van de Kamp's)	8½-oz. serving	530
TOSTADA SHELL (Old El Paso)	1 shell	55
TOTAL, cereal (General Mills)	1 cup (1 oz.)	110
TRIPE, canned (Libby's)	6-oz. serving	290
TRIPLE SEC LIQUEUR (Mr. Boston)	1 fl. oz.	79
TRIX, cereal (General Mills)	1 cup	110
TROPICAL CITRUS DRINK, chilled or *frozen (Five Alive)	6 fl. oz.	85
*TROPICAL QUENCHER DRINK, mix, dietetic, *Crystal Light*	8 fl. oz.	3
TUNA:		
Canned in oil:		
(Bumble Bee):		
Chunk, light, solids & liq.	½ cup	265
Solid, white, solids & liq.	½ cup	285
(Carnation) solids & liq.	6½-oz. can	427
(Progresso) light, solid	⅓ cup	150
(Sea Trader) chunk, light, solids & liq.	3¼ oz.	230
Canned in water:		
(Breast O'Chicken)	6½-oz. can	211
(Bumble Bee):		
Chunk, light, solids & liq.	½ cup	117
Solid, white, solids & liq.	½ cup	126
(Featherweight) light, chunk	6½-oz. can	210
(Sea Trader) white albacore	2 oz.	100
*TUNA HELPER (General Mills):		
Au gratin	⅓ pkg.	280

Food and Description	*Measure or Quantity*	*Calories*
Cold salad	⅕ pkg.	440
Buttery rice	⅕ pkg.	280
Creamy mushroom	⅕ pkg.	220
Creamy noodle or fettucini alfredo	⅕ pkg.	300
Tuna pot pie	⅙ pkg.	420
Tuna tetrazzini	⅕ pkg.	240
TUNA NOODLE CASSEROLE, frozen (Stouffer's)	10-oz. meal	310
TUNA PIE, frozen (Banquet)	8-oz. pie	395
TUNA SALAD:		
Home recipe	4-oz. serving	193
Canned (Carnation)	¼ of 7½-oz. can	100
TURF & SURF DINNER, frozen (Armour) *Classic Lights*	10-oz. meal	250
TURKEY:		
Fresh, roasted:		
Flesh & skin	4-oz. serving	253
Dark meat	2½" × 1⅝" × ¼" slice	43
Light meat	4" × 2" × ¼" slice	75
Barbecued (Louis Rich) breast, half	1 oz.	40
Packaged:		
(Carl Buddig):		
Regular	1 oz.	50
Ham or salami	1 oz.	40
Hebrew National, breast	1 oz.	37
(Hormel) breast	1 slice	30
(Louis Rich):		
Turkey bologna	1-oz. slice	60
Turkey cotto salami	1-oz. slice	50
Turkey ham, chopped	1-oz. slice	45
Turkey pastrami	1-oz. slice	35
(Ohse):		
Oven cooked	1 oz.	30
Turkey bologna	1 oz.	70
Turkey salami	1 oz.	50
(Oscar Mayer) breast, oven roasted	.7-oz. slice	23
(Smok-A-Roma) breast	1-oz. slice	30
Smoked (Louis Rich):		
Drumsticks	1 oz. (without bone)	40
Wing drumettes	1 oz. (without bone)	45

Food and Description	Measure or Quantity	Calories
TURKEY DINNER OR ENTREE, frozen:		
(Armour) *Dinner Classics*	11½-oz. meal	320
(Banquet)	10½-oz. dinner	390
(Budget Gourmet):		
Dinner, breast, stuffed	11-oz. meal	230
Entree:		
Regular, a la king, with rice	10-oz. meal	390
Light, glazed	9-oz. meal	270
Slim Selects, glazed	9-oz. meal	270
(Healthy Choice) breast	10½-oz. meal	290
(Le Menu) healthy style, sliced	10-oz. dinner	210
(Stouffer's):		
Regular, tetrazzini	10-oz. meal	380
Lean Cuisine, Dijon	9½-oz. meal	270
Right Course, sliced, in curry sauce with rice pilaf	8⅜-oz. meal	320
(Swanson):		
Regular	11½-oz. dinner	350
Homestyle Recipe	9-oz. entree	290
Hungry Man	17-oz. dinner	550
(Weight Watchers) stuffed, breast	8½-oz. meal	260
TURKEY NUGGET, frozen (Empire Kosher)	¼ of 12-oz. pkg.	255
TURKEY PATTY, frozen (Empire Kosher)	¼ of 12-oz. pkg.	188
TURKEY PIE, frozen:		
(Banquet)	7-oz. pie	510
(Empire Kosher)	8-oz. pie	491
(Morton)	7-oz. pie	420
(Stouffer's)	10-oz. pie	540
(Swanson) regular	7-oz. pie	380
TURKEY TETRAZZINI, frozen:		
(Stouffer's)	6-oz. serving	240
(Weight Watchers)	10-oz. pkg.	310
TURNIP GREENS, canned (Allen's) chopped, solids & liq.	½ cup	20
TURNIP ROOTS, frozen (McKenzie) diced	1 oz.	4
TURNOVER:		
Frozen (Pepperidge Farm):		
Apple	1 turnover	300
Blueberry, peach or raspberry	1 turnover	310
Refrigerated (Pillsbury)	1 turnover	170

Food and Description	Measure or Quantity	Calories

U

Food and Description	Measure or Quantity	Calories
ULTRA DIET QUICK (TKI Foods):		
Bar	1.2-oz. bar	130
*Mix:		
Dutch chocolate made with low-fat milk	8 fl. oz.	200
Strawberry delight or vanilla creme	8 fl. oz.	100
ULTRA SLIM FAST:		
Canned:		
Chocolate royale	11 fl. oz.	230
French Vanilla	11 fl. oz.	210
Mix:		
Regular:		
Cafe Mocha	1 scoop	100
*Cafe Mocha	8 fl. oz.	200
Chocolate Fantasy	1 scoop	120
*Chocolate Fantasy	8 fl. oz.	250
Chocolate malt	1 scoop	100
*Chocolate malt	8 fl. oz.	190
French vanilla	1 scoop	100
*French vanilla	8 fl. oz.	190
Fruit juice	1 scoop	90
*Fruit juice	8 fl. oz.	200
Strawberry supreme	1 scoop	100
*Strawberry supreme	8 fl. oz.	190
Plus:		
Chocolate Fantasy	1 scoop	120
*Chocolate Fantasy	8 fl. oz.	250
Vanilla creme	1 scoop	110
*Vanilla creme	8 fl. oz.	240

Food and Description	Measure or Quantity	Calories

V

Food and Description	Measure or Quantity	Calories
VALPOLICELLA WINE (Antinori)	3 fl. oz.	84
VANDERMINT, liqueur	1 fl. oz.	90
VANILLA EXTRACT		
(Virginia Dare)	1 tsp.	10
VEAL, broiled, medium cooked:		
Loin chop	4 oz.	265
Rib, roasted	4 oz.	305
Steak or cutlet, lean & fat	4 oz.	245
VEAL DINNER, frozen:		
(Armour) *Dinner Classics,* parmigiana	11¼-oz. meal	400
(Le Menu) parmigiana	11½-oz. dinner	390
(Morton) parmigiana	10-oz. dinner	260
(Swanson) parmigiana, *Hungry Man*	18¼-oz. dinner	590
(Weight Watchers) parmigiana, patty	8.4-oz. meal	220
VEAL STEAK, frozen (Hormel):		
Regular	4-oz. serving	130
Breaded	4-oz. serving	240
VEGETABLE BOUILLON		
(Herb-Ox):		
Cube	1 cube	6
Packet	1 packet	12
VEGETABLE JUICE COCKTAIL:		
Regular:		
(Mott's)	6 fl. oz.	30
(Smucker's)	8 fl. oz.	58
V-8	6 fl. oz.	35
Dietetic:		
(S&W) *Nutradiet,* low sodium	6 fl. oz.	35
V-8, low sodium	6 fl. oz.	35
VEGETABLES, MIXED:		
Canned, regular pack:		
(A&P)	½ cup	45
(La Choy) drained:		
Chinese	⅓ of 14-oz. pkg.	12
Chop Suey	½ cup	9
(Pathmark)	½ cup	35

Food and Description	Measure or Quantity	Calories
(Town House)	½ cup	45
(Veg-All)	½ cup	35
Canned, dietetic pack:		
(Featherweight)	½ cup	40
(Larsen) *Fresh-Lite*	½ cup	35
Frozen:		
(A&P):		
California blend	3.3 oz.	25
Italian style	3.3 oz.	40
Oriental style	3.3 oz.	25
Stew	4 oz.	60
Winter blend	3.3 oz.	24
(Bel-Air):		
Regular	3.3 oz.	65
Hawaiian	3.3 oz.	50
Rancho fiesta	3.3 oz.	70
Winter mix	3.3 oz.	40
(Birds Eye):		
Regular:		
Broccoli, cauliflower & carrots in cheese sauce	5 oz.	100
Carrots, peas & onions, deluxe	⅓ pkg.	52
Medley, in butter sauce	⅓ of 10-oz. pkg.	62
Farm Fresh:		
Broccoli, cauliflower & carrot strips	3.2 oz.	25
Brussels sprouts, cauliflower & carrots	3.2 oz.	30
Stir Fry, Chinese style	⅓ pkg.	35
(Chun King) chow mein, drained	4 oz.	32
(Frosty Acres):		
Regular	3.3 oz.	65
Dutch	3.2 oz.	30
Oriental	3.2 oz.	25
Soup mix	3 oz.	45
Stew	3 oz.	42
Swiss mix	3 oz.	25
(Green Giant):		
Regular:		
Broccoli, cauliflower & carrots in cheese sauce	½ cup	60
Corn, broccoli bounty	½ cup	60
Harvest Fresh	½ cup	60
Harvest Get Togethers:		
Broccoli-cauliflower medley	½ cup	60
Broccoli fanfare	½ cup	80

Food and Description	Measure or Quantity	Calories
(Health Valley)	½ cup	68
(La Choy) stir fry	4 oz.	40
(Larsen):		
Regular or chuckwagon blend	3.3 oz.	70
California blend or Italian		
blend	3.3 oz.	30
Oriental blend	3.3 oz.	25
(Ore-Ida):		
Medley, breaded	3 oz.	160
Stew vegetables	3 oz.	60
(Southland):		
Gumbo	⅕ of 16-oz. pkg.	40
Stew	4 oz.	60
VEGETABLE STEW, canned *Dinty Moore* (Hormel)	7½-oz. serving	170
"VEGETARIAN FOODS":		
Canned or dry:		
Chicken, fried (Loma Linda) with gravy	1½-oz. piece	70
Chili (Worthington)	½ cup	177
Choplet (Worthington)	1 choplet	50
Dinner cuts (Loma Linda) drained	1 piece	60
Dinner loaf (Loma Linda)	¼ cup	50
Franks, big (Loma Linda)	1.9-oz. frank	100
Franks, sizzle (Loma Linda)	2.2-oz. frank	85
FriChik (Worthington)	1 piece	75
Little links (Loma Linda) drained	.8-oz. link	40
Non-meatballs (Worthington)	1 meatball	32
Nuteena (Loma Linda)	½" slice	160
Patty mix (Loma Linda)	¼ cup	50
Prime Stakes	1 slice	171
Proteena (Loma Linda)	½" slice	140
Sandwich spread (Loma Linda)	1 T.	23
*Soyagen, all purpose powder (Loma Linda)	1 cup	130
Soyameal, any kind (Worthington)	1 oz.	120
Soyameat (Worthington):		
Beef, sliced	1 slice	44
Chicken, diced	1 oz.	40
Stew pack (Loma Linda) drained	2 oz.	70
Super links (Worthington)	1 link	110
Swiss steak with gravy (Loma Linda)	1 steak	140
Vega-links (Worthington)	1 link	55
Vegelona (Loma Linda)	½" slice	100

Food and Description	Measure or Quantity	Calories
Wheat protein	4 oz.	124
Worthington 209	1 slice	58
Frozen:		
Beef pie (Worthington)	1 pie	278
Bologna (Loma Linda)	1 oz.	75
Chicken, fried (Loma Linda)	2-oz. serving	180
Chic-Ketts (Worthington)	1 oz.	53
Corned beef, sliced (Worthington)	1 slice	32
Fri Pats (Worthington)	1 patty	204
Meatballs (Loma Linda)	1 meatball	63
Meatless salami (Worthington)	1 slice	44
Prosage (Worthington)	1 link	60
Smoked beef, slices (Worthington)	1 slice	14
Wham, roll (Worthington)	1 slice	36
VERMOUTH:		
Dry & extra dry (Lejon; Noilly Pratt)	1 fl. oz.	33
Sweet (Lejon; Taylor)	1 fl. oz.	45
VICHY WATER (Schweppes)	Any quantity	0
VINEGAR, DISTILLED OR CIDER	1 T.	2
VODKA (See DISTILLED LIQUOR)		

Food and Description	Measure or Quantity	Calories

W

WAFFLE, frozen: (See also
  PANCAKE & WAFFLE MIX):
  (Aunt Jemima):

Original	2½-oz. waffle	173
Apple cinnamon	2½-oz. waffle	176
Blueberry	2½-oz. waffle	175
Oat bran	2½-oz. waffle	154
(Downyflake):		
Plain	1 waffle	60
Blueberry	1 waffle	90
Buttermilk	1 waffle	95
Jumbo	1 waffle	85
Rice bran	1 waffle	105
(Eggo):		
Regular:		
Apple cinnamon or blueberry	1 waffle	130
Buttermilk or homestyle	1 waffle	120
Common Sense, oat bran, with		
fruit & nut	1 waffle	120
Nutri-Grain, plain or raisin &		
bran	1 waffle	130
(Weight Watchers) Belgian	1½ oz.	120
WAFFLE BREAKFAST, frozen		
(Swanson) *Great Starts*:		
Regular, with bacon	2.2 oz.	230
Belgian, & sausage	2.85 oz.	280
WALNUT, English or Persian		
(Diamond A)	1 cup	679
WALNUT FLAVORING, black,		
imitation (Durkee)	1 tsp.	4
WATER CHESTNUT, canned:		
(Chun King) whole, drained	½ of 8½-oz. can	85
(La Choy) drained	¼ cup	16
WATERCRESS, trimmed	½ cup	3
WATERMELON:		
Wedge	4" × 8" wedge	111
Diced	½ cup	21

Food and Description	Measure or Quantity	Calories
WELSH RAREBIT:		
Home recipe	1 cup	415
Canned (Snow's)	½ cup	170
Frozen:		
(Green Giant)	5-oz. serving	219
(Stouffer's)	5-oz. serving	350
WENDY'S RESTAURANT:		
Bacon, breakfast	1 strip	55
Bacon cheeseburger on white bun	1 serving	460
Breakfast sandwich	1 sandwich	370
Buns:		
Wheat, multi-grain	1 bun	135
White	1 bun	160
Chicken sandwich on multi-grain bun	1 sandwich	320
Chili:		
Regular	8 oz.	260
Large	12 oz.	390
Condiments:		
Bacon	½ strip	30
Cheese, American	1 slice	70
Onion rings	.3-oz. piece	4
Pickle, dill	4 slices	1
Relish	.3-oz. serving	14
Tomato	1 slice	2
Danish	1 piece	360
Drinks:		
Coffee	6 fl. oz.	2
Cola:		
Regular	12 fl. oz	110
Dietetic	12 fl. oz.	Tr.
Fruit flavored drink	12 fl. oz.	110
Hot chocolate	6 fl. oz.	100
Milk:		
Regular	8 fl. oz.	150
Chocolate	8 fl. oz.	210
Non-cola	12 fl. oz.	100
Orange juice	6 fl. oz.	80
Egg, scrambled	1 order	190
Frosty dairy dessert:		
Small	12 fl. oz.	400
Medium	16 fl. oz.	533
Large	20 fl. oz.	667
Hamburger:		
Double, on white bun	1 serving	560
Kids Meal	1 serving	220

Food and Description	Measure or Quantity	Calories
Single:		
On wheat bun	1 serving	340
On white bun	1 serving	350
Omelet:		
Ham & cheese	1 omelet	250
Ham, cheese & mushroom	1 omelet	290
Mushroom, onion & green pepper	1 omelet	210
Potato:		
Baked, hot stuffed:		
Plain	1 potato	250
Broccoli & cheese	1 potato	500
Cheese	1 potato	590
Chicken á la King	1 potato	350
Sour cream & chives	1 potato	460
Stroganoff & sour cream	1 potato	490
French fries	regular order	280
Home fries	1 order	360
Salad Bar, *Garden Spot:*		
Alfalfa sprouts	2 oz.	20
Bacon bits	⅛ oz.	10
Blueberries, fresh	1 T.	8
Breadstick	1 piece	20
Broccoli	½ cup	14
Cantaloupe	1 piece (2 oz.)	4
Carrot	¼ cup	12
Cauliflower	½ cup	14
Cheese:		
American, imitation	1 oz.	70
Cheddar, imitation	1 oz.	90
Cottage	½ cup	110
Mozzarella, imitation	1 oz.	90
Swiss, imitation	1 oz.	80
Chow mein noodles	¼ cup	60
Coleslaw	½ cup	90
Crouton	1 piece	2
Cucumber	¼ cup	4
Mushroom	¼ cup	6
Onions, red	1 T.	4
Orange, fresh	1 piece	5
Pasta salad	½ cup	134
Peaches, in syrup	1 piece	8
Peas, green	½ cup	60
Peppers:		
Banana or mild pepperoncini	1 T.	18
Bell	¼ cup	4
Jalapeño	1 T.	9
Pineapple chunks in juice	½ cup	80

Food and Description	Measure or Quantity	Calories
Tomato	1 oz.	6
Turkey ham	¼ cup	46
Watermelon, fresh	1 piece (1 oz.)	1
Salad dressing:		
Regular:		
Blue cheese	1 T.	60
French, red	1 T.	70
Italian, golden	1 T.	45
Oil	1 T.	130
Ranch	1 T.	80
1000 Island	1 T.	70
Dietetic:		
Bacon & tomato	1 T.	45
Cucumber, creamy	1 T.	50
Italian	1 T.	25
1000 Island	1 T.	45
Wine vinegar	1 T.	2
Salad, side, pick-up window	1 salad	110
Salad, taco	1 salad	390
Sausage	1 patty	200
Toast: Regular, with margarine	1 slice	125
French	1 slice	200
WESTERN DINNER, frozen:		
(Banquet)	11-oz. dinner	630
(Morton) regular	10-oz. dinner	290
(Swanson) *Hungry Man*	17¾-oz. dinner	820
WHEAT GERM CEREAL		
(Kretschmer)	¼ cup (1 oz.)	110
WHEAT GERM, RAW (Elam's)	1 T.	28
WHEAT HEARTS, cereal		
(General Mills)	1 oz. (3½ T.)	110
WHEATIES, cereal	1 cup (1 oz.)	100
WHISKEY SOUR COCKTAIL		
(Mr. Boston)	3 fl. oz.	120
***WHISKEY SOUR MIX**		
(Bar-Tender's)	3½ fl. oz.	177
WHITE CASTLE:		
Bun only	.9-oz. bun	74
Cheese only	1 piece	31
Cheeseburger	1 sandwich	200
Chicken sandwich	1 sandwich	186
Fish sandwich	1 sandwich	155
French fries	1 order	301
Hamburger	1 sandwich	161
Onion chips	1 order	329
Onion rings	1 order	245
Sausage & egg sandwich	1 sandwich	322

Food and Description	Measure or Quantity	Calories
Sausage sandwich	1 sandwich	196
WHITEFISH, LAKE:		
Baked, stuffed	4 oz.	244
Smoked	4 oz.	176
WIENER WRAP (Pillsbury)	1 piece	60
WILD BERRY DRINK,		
canned (Hi-C)	6 fl. oz.	92
WINE (See specific type, such as CHIANTI; SHERRY; etc.)		
WINE, COOKING (Holland House):		
Marsala	1 fl. oz.	9
Red	1 fl. oz.	6
Sherry	1 fl. oz.	5
Vermouth or white	1 fl. oz.	1
WINE COOLER (Bartles & Jaymes):		
Light berry	6 fl. oz.	71
Premium berry, premium peach or premium red sangria	6 fl. oz.	107
Premium black cherry	6 fl. oz.	104
Premium original	6 fl. oz.	99

Food and Description	Measure or Quantity	Calories

Y

YEAST, BAKER'S (Fleischmann's):		
Dry, active	1 packet	20
Fresh & household, active	.6-oz. cake	15
YOGURT:		
Regular:		
Plain:		
(Borden) *Lite-Line*	8-oz. container	140
(Columbo) lite	8-oz. container	110
(Dannon):		
Low-fat	8-oz. cont.	110
Non-fat	8-oz. cont.	140
(Friendship)	8-oz. container	150
(Johanna Farms)	8-oz. container	150
(Lucerne):		
Gourmet	6-oz. container	130
Lowfat	8-oz. container	160
(Weight Watchers) non-fat	8-oz. container	150
Yoplait, regular	6-oz. container	130
Apple (Dannon) Dutch, Fruit-on-the-Bottom	8-oz. container	240
Apple & raisins (Whitney's)	6-oz. container	200
Apricot (Lucerne) lowfat	8-oz. container	260
Apricot-pineapple (Lucerne) lowfat	8-oz. container	260
Banana:		
(Dannon) Fruit-on-the-Bottom	8-oz. container	240
(Lucerne) lowfat	8-oz. container	260
Yoplait, regular	6-oz. container	190
Blueberry:		
(Dannon) *Fresh Flavors*	8-oz. container	200
(Lucerne):		
Gourmet	6-oz. container	190
Nonfat	8-oz. container	180
(Mountain High)	8-oz. container	220
(Sweet 'n Low)	8-oz. container	150
Yoplait, custard style	6-oz. container	190

Food and Description	Measure or Quantity	Calories
Blueberry (Columbo) lite	8-oz. container	190
Boysenberry:		
(Dannon) Fruit-on-the-Bottom	8-oz. container	240
(Sweet 'n Low)	8-oz. container	150
Cherry:		
(Breyers) black	8-oz. container	270
(Dannon) Fruit-on-the-Bottom	8-oz. container	240
(Lucerne) nonfat	8-oz. container	180
(Sweet 'n Low)	8-oz. container	150
Yoplait:		
Breakfast yogurt, with almonds	6-oz. container	200
Custard style	6-oz. container	180
Light	6-oz. container	90
Cherry-vanilla (Borden) Lite-Line	8-oz. container	240
Coffee:		
(Colombo) lite	8-oz. container	190
(Dannon)	8-oz. container	200
(Friendship)	8-oz. container	210
(Johanna Farms)	8-oz. container	220
Exotic fruit (Dannon) Fruit-on-the-Bottom	8-oz. container	240
Lemon:		
(Dannon) Fresh Flavors	8-oz. container	200
(Johanna Farms)	8-oz.container	220
(Lucerne) lowfat	8-oz. container	260
(Sweet'n Low)	8-oz. container	150
Yoplait:		
Regular	6-oz. container	190
Custard style	6-oz. container	190
Lime (Lucerne) lowfat	8-oz. container	260
Mixed berries (Dannon):		
Extra Smooth	4.4-oz. container	130
Fruit-on-the-Bottom	8-oz. container	240
Orange, Yoplait	6-oz. container	190
Peach:		
(Borden) Lite-Line	8-oz. container	230
(Colombo) lite	8-oz. container	190
(Dannon) Fruit-on-the-Bottom	8-oz. container	240
(Friendship)	8-oz. container	240
(Lucerne) gourmet	6-oz. container	190
(Sweet'n Low)	8-oz. container	150
Yoplait:		
Regular	6-oz. container	190
Light	6-oz. container	90
Peach melba (Lucerne)	8-oz. container	260

Food and Description	Measure or Quantity	Calories
Peach pecan (Lucerne)	6-oz. container	190
Piña colada:		
(Dannon) Fruit-on-the-Bottom	8-oz. container	240
(Friendship)	8-oz. container	230
Yoplait, custard style	6-oz. container	190
Pineapple:		
(Breyers)	8-oz. container	270
(Light n' Lively)	8-oz. container	240
(Lucerne)	8-oz. container	260
Yoplait	6-oz. container	190
Raspberry:		
(Breyers) red	8-oz. container	260
(Dannon):		
Extra Smooth	4.4-oz. container	130
Fresh Flavors	8-oz. container	200
(Light n' Lively) red	8-oz. container	230
(Lucerne) regular	8-oz. container	260
(Sweet 'n Low)	8-oz container	150
Yoplait:		
Regular	6-oz. container	190
Custard style	6-oz. container	190
Light	6-oz. container	90
Strawberry:		
(Borden) *Lite-Line*	8-oz. container	240
(Columbo) lite	8-oz. container	190
(Dannon) *Fresh Flavors*	8-oz. container	200
(Friendship)	8-oz. container	230
(Light n' Lively)	8-oz. container	240
(Lucerne):		
Gourmet	6-oz. container	190
Nonfat	8-oz. container	180
Yoplait, light	6-oz. container	90
Strawberry-banana (Light n' Lively)	8-oz. container	260
Vanilla:		
(Breyers)	8-oz. container	230
(Columbo) lite	8-oz. container	110
(Dannon) light, regular or cherry	8-oz. container	100
(Friendship)	8-oz. container	210
(Lucerne) lowfat	8-oz. container	260
Yoplait, custard style	6-oz. container	180
Frozen:		
Hard:		
Chocolate (Häagen-Dazs)	3 fl. oz.	130
Mocha Swiss almond (Colombo) gourmet	3 fl. oz.	120

Food and Description	Measure or Quantity	Calories
Peach:		
(Breyers)	½ cup	110
(Häagen-Dazs)	3 fl. oz.	120
Peanut butter cup (Columbo) gourmet	3 fl. oz.	140
Strawberry:		
(Breyers)	½ cup	110
(Häagen-Dazs)	3 fl. oz.	120
Strawberry-banana (Breyers)	½ cup	110
Vanilla:		
(Breyers)	½ cup	120
(Häagen-Dazs)	3 fl. oz.	130
Soft (Dannon):		
Blueberry, cappuccino, cheesecake, lemon meringue, piña colada or strawberry	½ cup	100
Chocolate	½ cup	120
YOGURT BAR, frozen:		
(Baskin-Robbins):		
Dutch chocolate chip	1 bar	260
Praline vanilla	1 bar	250
(Dannon):		
Bars, *Danny:*		
Plain, uncoated:		
Chocolate or vanilla	1 bar	60
Piña colada	1 bar	70
Carob-coated, boysenberry	1 bar	140
Chocolate-coated, any flavor	1 bar	130
On A Stick, all flavors	1¾-oz. piece	50
(TCBY—The Country's Best Yogurt)		
Yog-a-Bar:		
Toasted almonds	1 bar	240
Vanilla:		
With heath	1 bar	220
Low fat	1 bar	170
Sugar free	1 bar	120
YOGURT DRINK		
(Dannon) all flavors	8 oz.	190
(Weight Watchers) frozen, chocolate	7½ oz.	220

Food and Description	Measure or Quantity	Calories

Z

ZINFANDEL WINE (Louis M. Martini) regular vintage   3 fl. oz.   64

ZINGERS (Dolly Madison):

Devils food	1¼-oz. piece	140
Raspberry	1¼-oz. piece	130

ZWEIBACK (Gerber; Nabisco)   1 piece   30